Ruttonjee Sanatorium

Life And Times

Michael Humphries

© Michael Humphries 1996

All rights reserved

ISBN 978-1495342578

Design & layout by Step Design Consultants

Printed by Wing Yiu Printing Company

Cover Illustration: The buildings of the Ruttonjee Sanatorium in Wanchai were formerly those of the Royal Naval Hospital in Hong Kong, as pictured here in the Illustrated London News of September 27th 1873. The original site was a bluff peninsula projecting into Hong Kong harbour. Kellet's Island can be seen in the distance; much of the harbour has since been reclaimed. In the centre foreground, three stone nullahs can be seen. Although the nullahs no longer exist, the street is now known as Stone Nullah Lane.

The publication of this book is sponsored by
Ruttonjee Estates Continuation Limited,
Ms. Vera Ruttonjee-Desai and
Mr. Rusy M. Shroff, MBE.

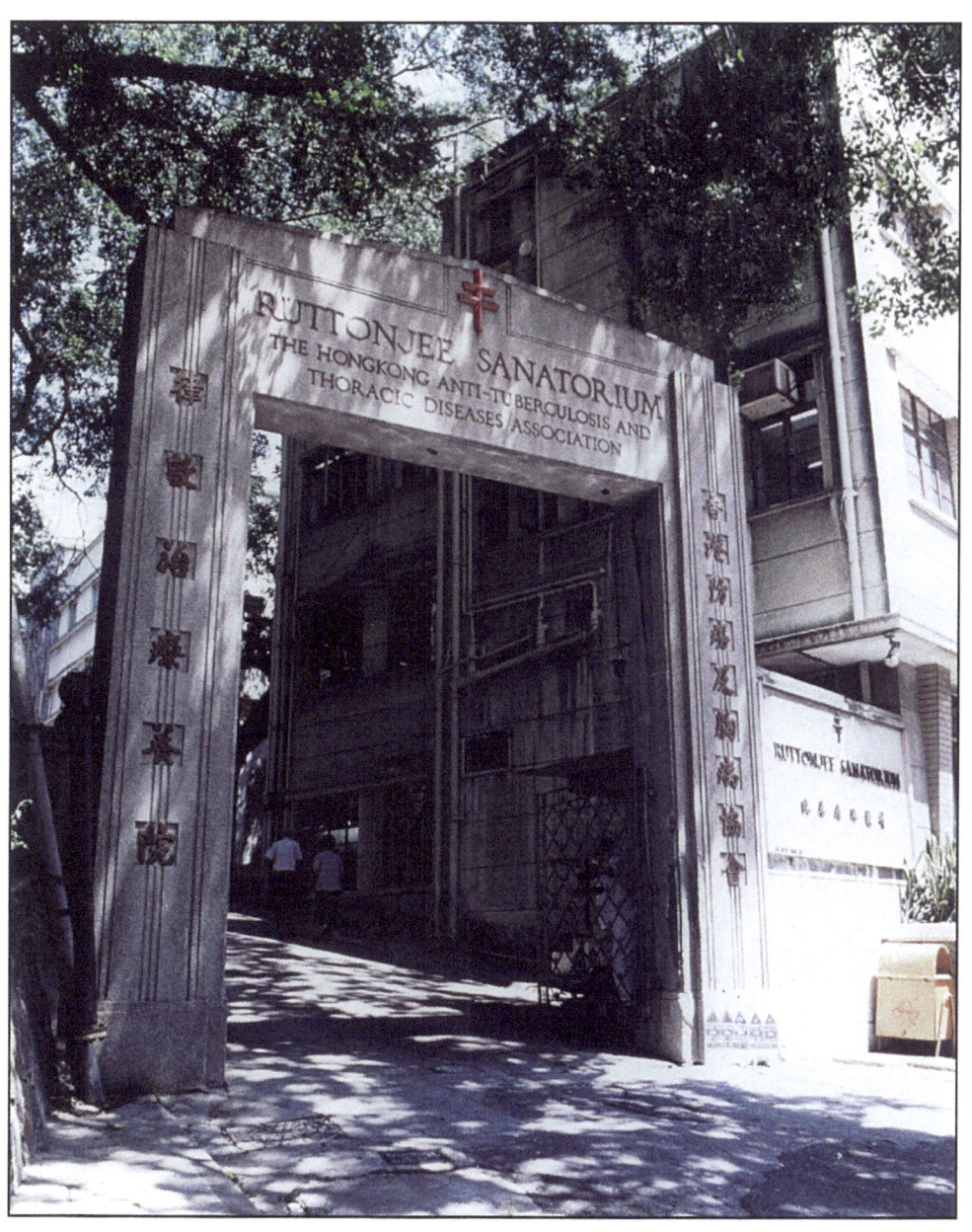

The original stone gateway to Ruttonjee Sanatorium.

We knew how to cure TB, but we dropped the ball by not ensuring proper treatment.

We have squandered a precious legacy.

Dr. Michael Iseman 1993

It seems almost incredible that during this century and the previous one,
a single disease, tuberculosis, was responsible for the deaths of approximately
one thousand million human beings.

Dr. Frank Ryan 1992
Tuberculosis: The greatest story never told

Acknowledgements

I would like to thank the following for their invaluable contributions to the research and publication of this book.

The Columban Sisters, particularly Sister Mary Gabriel; The Board of Directors of the Hong Kong Tuberculosis, Chest and Heart Diseases Association, and the General Secretary Mr. James Yue; The Reverend Carl Smith, who provided the greatest part of the research on the early history of the Seamen's and Royal Naval Hospital; Mr. Choi Chi-Cheung and Dr. Lau Yun-Woo of the Hong Kong Public Records Office; Ms. Joffree Chan and Ms. Ang Yee of the Hong Kong Museum of History; Mr. Alan Reid, Honorary Archivist of Jardine Matheson and Co., and Ms. Elaine Ho of Jardine Danby Ltd. gave welcome advice on sources of historical material.

I am also grateful to Professor G. H. Choa for reviewing the text and Dr. Robert Teoh and Dr. Raymond Lasserre for their enthusiastic support and encouragement. Sincerest thanks to Mr. Douglas Bertram for allowing reproduction of rare and precious photographs of the Royal Naval Hospital. Mrs. Winnie Chang and Mrs. Zoe Chan provided valuable advice. Special thanks are due to Mr. Stephen Barry and Ms. Stella Han for creative ideas and the layout of text and photographs.

Photographs have been reproduced by permission of the Urban Council of Hong Kong Museum of Art (pages 4, 6, 7, 16). The photograph on page 2 was taken by Mr. Michael Chung, courtesy of Joan Boivin Photography. The map on page 10 is reproduced with permission of the Director of Lands, Hong Kong Government. Sincere thanks to Mr. John Fox for editing the manuscript and also to Mr. Tom Brand and Pat Elliott Shircore for helpful comments.

Finally, I am indebted to Mr. R. M. Shroff MBE, Chairman of the Board of Directors of the Hong Kong Tuberculosis, Chest and Heart Diseases Association for contributing the chapters entitled "The Ruttonjee Family" and "The Founding of the Hong Kong Anti-Tuberculosis Association".

For Rose and Emma

Contents

Preface	1
Introduction	3
Historical Perspectives	7
Medicine in the South China Region	9
The Seamen's Hospital 1843-1873	11
The Royal Naval Hospital 1873-1942	17
The Ruttonjee Family	21
The Founding of the Hong Kong Anti-Tuberculosis Association	23
Ruttonjee Sanatorium 1949-1991	25
Contributions to the Fight Against Tuberculosis	31
Sister Mary Aquinas	37
Sister Mary Gabriel	41
The Ruttonjee Hospital	43
Bibliography	45
Appendices	53

Preface

The Ruttonjee Sanatorium served as a specialist centre for the treatment of tuberculosis from 1949 until 1991, inclusive. The core of the original building was erected as the Seamen's Hospital in 1843 and, after reconstruction, became the Royal Naval Hospital in 1873. The buildings occupied an attractive site on a peninsula within Hong Kong harbour with panoramic views over Kowloon. At the East Gate of the hospital a set of steps leading into the sea allowed sailors to be taken directly from their ships to the hospital by small boats. With reclamation, the site gradually became surrounded by buildings and cut off from the sea. After the Second World War, the building was refurbished and re-named the Ruttonjee Sanatorium, accommodating nearly 400 patients with tuberculosis and other respiratory diseases. However, the original buildings deteriorated and were demolished in 1992.

The idea behind this book arose in 1987 when quite by chance I came across a print hanging on the wall of an antique shop in Stanley. It was a picture from the Illustrated London News of September 27th 1873 of the Royal Naval Hospital in Hong Kong, yet was instantly recognisable as the Ruttonjee Sanatorium, where I happened to be working at the time as Medical Officer. The site, building, trees and even the flagpole hardly appeared to have changed for more than 100 years. It was then that I started to research the background of the hospital, a task that assumed increasing urgency as the buildings were soon to be demolished.

The more facts and figures that were unearthed, the more exciting the project appeared. It soon became apparent that the history of the Ruttonjee Sanatorium is a remarkable one, being inextricably linked with two outstanding phenomena; the history of Hong Kong itself, and tuberculosis, one of mankind's greatest afflictions. Many of the events and developments of the site of the Sanatorium are a reflection of the turbulent history of Hong Kong.

The Sanatorium had established an international reputation for research and education in tuberculosis, having been administered throughout its 40 years of life by a community of remarkable and dedicated professionals, the Columban Sisters. Only after detailed research in the library did the full extent of the contributions to the research and control of tuberculosis become obvious. My purpose in writing this small book is to document that special contribution.

But as always, times must change. The old building deteriorated and was demolished, and the Sisters gradually retired or moved to other activities where there was a more urgent need for their care and expertise.

A modern district hospital, the Ruttonjee Hospital, has been built on the site of the original Sanatorium, and was opened by the Governor of Hong Kong, the Right Honourable Christopher Patten, on April 22nd 1994. The new hospital will care for patients with a broad range of medical conditions, including tuberculosis and respiratory diseases, to continue the Ruttonjee tradition of care for the people of Hong Kong.

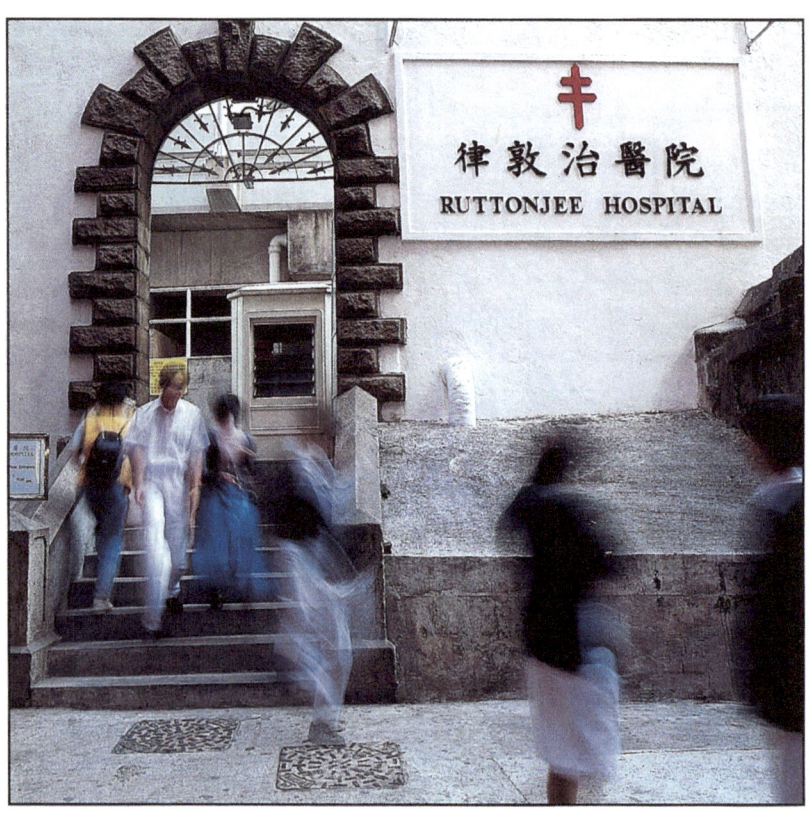

The East Gate of the Seamen's Hospital used to receive ill sailors from small boats, as the sea reached the foot of the gate. Currently the gate opens onto a busy market in Wanchai Road.

Introduction

Hong Kong was first claimed by Sir George Bremer on January 26th 1841. A matshed hospital was one of the earliest buildings erected but it was destroyed by a typhoon, and this event prompted builders to design and create more robust structures that could withstand the ravages of nature. The building of the Seamen's Hospital started in 1842 and the first patients were admitted in 1843, an early example of government and commerce coming together to provide services for the community. The subsequent sale of the building to the Royal Navy in 1873 was presumably a relief to many sailors, who previously had to endure almost intolerable discomfort on hospital ships, whose environment alone was responsible for the premature death of many seamen. In subsequent years, the Royal Naval Hospital was witness to the many vagaries of the Hong Kong climate, including the deadly typhoon of 1874 and numerous landslips from the site into adjoining Wanchai.

The staff and patients endured very difficult conditions during the invasion and subsequent occupation by the Japanese in 1941. After the Second World War, social deprivation, malnutrition and mass migration brought tuberculosis in its wake and the challenge to alleviate the suffering and control the illness was taken up by Mr. J. H. Ruttonjee and other founder members of the Hong Kong Anti-Tuberculosis Association. The Royal Navy abandoned their badly damaged hospital, but the buildings soon acquired a new purpose, and a new name; the Ruttonjee Sanatorium. The Sanatorium opened in 1949, however, it was two decades before the downward trend in tuberculosis notifications in Hong Kong could be described as satisfactory.

The 1980's witnessed a steady decline in the numbers of patients with tuberculosis and, together with an emphasis on outpatient treatment and increasing demands from other areas of healthcare, the old Sanatorium had served its purpose and was demolished in 1992. The new Ruttonjee Hospital was built in its place in the garden of the original site. The new hospital not only cares for patients with tuberculosis and respiratory diseases, but also houses general medical and surgical facilities, and a geriatric unit. Hence the growth and development of the hospital site from 1842 to the present day has mirrored the changing social structure and healthcare needs of the population of Hong Kong.

From 1949 until 1988, the Columban Sisters provided administrative, medical and nursing expertise to the Sanatorium. The Sisters led a loyal and hard-working staff, many of whom worked at the Sanatorium for many years, even decades. Within this environment, a number of important research findings were made, and the Sanatorium earned an international reputation for teaching and clinical care.

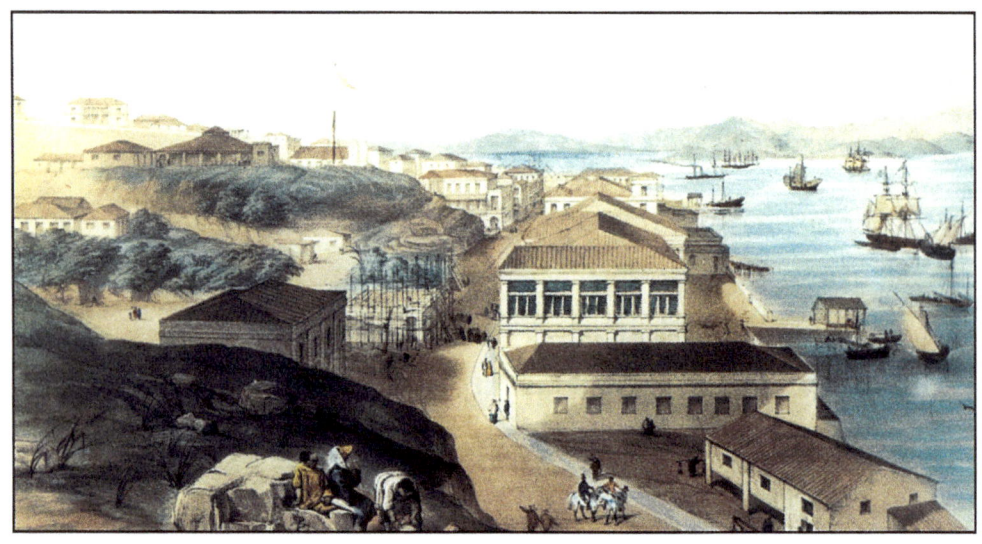

View of Queen's Road and the harbour looking West from the Seamen's Hospital.

These achievements were made possible by the vision and leadership of remarkable people. Sister Mary Aquinas earned a worldwide reputation for lecturing in tuberculosis based on scientific principles, extraordinary clinical experience and much common sense. Sister Mary Gabriel earned acclaim for clinical research in such varied areas as asthma and mite allergy, immunology, side effects of anti-tuberculosis drugs, tuberculous meningitis and palliative care of the terminally ill. Indeed the Sisters, together with dedicated nursing staff, were practising holistic medicine and palliative care from the early 1950's, which by Hong Kong standards was revolutionary. When the Society for the Promotion of Hospice Care was founded in Hong Kong, it was highly appropriate that their first home should be the Ruttonjee Sanatorium.

As an editorial in the Times of London recently pointed out, despite the frequent appearance of the consumptive hero or heroine in literature, there is nothing remotely romantic about tuberculosis. The disease wrecks previously healthy individuals and destroys life; in many countries the disease is running out of control with disastrous consequences, a situation that is exacerbated by the AIDS pandemic.

Throughout history, tuberculosis has been responsible for the deaths of more than 1000 million human beings. Currently, control of the disease is in a lamentable position and there is no reason to doubt that several hundred million people will perish from tuberculosis in the next 100 years. This situation prompted the World Health Organization, in 1993, to declare tuberculosis a global emergency. There will be 90 million new cases of tuberculosis between the years 1990 and 2000 worldwide and the disease will claim 30 million lives in that time. Much of this morbidity and mortality will be in Asia. In Hong Kong, tuberculosis has claimed nearly 150,000 lives since 1900. Fortunately, the disease has been on the decline in the territory since the late 1950's.

In a number of countries, including the United States of America and many African nations, there has been a resurgence in tuberculosis. The problem in many countries has been a lack of resources or the will to develop and maintain effective control measures. In Hong Kong we have been very fortunate to have enlightened individuals and a government with the determination and resources to treat tuberculosis properly, and follow up patients to ensure that no-one drops out of treatment through poor education or social disadvantage.

The Ruttonjee Sanatorium was very much part of this caring tradition and, together with the Hong Kong Government Chest Service, offered supervised anti-tuberculosis treatment and long-term care absolutely free of charge. Probably Hong Kong's greatest contribution to medicine worldwide has been to demonstrate that fully supervised treatment of tuberculosis with highly organized follow-up of patients can cure 95% of sufferers. It has also been demonstrated that acceptable and low-cost treatment schedules can be adapted to suit almost any patient's individual circumstances. Therefore the work of the Hong Kong Government Chest Service and hospitals such as the new Ruttonjee must go on and indeed intensify in order to protect future generations from the ravages of tuberculosis.

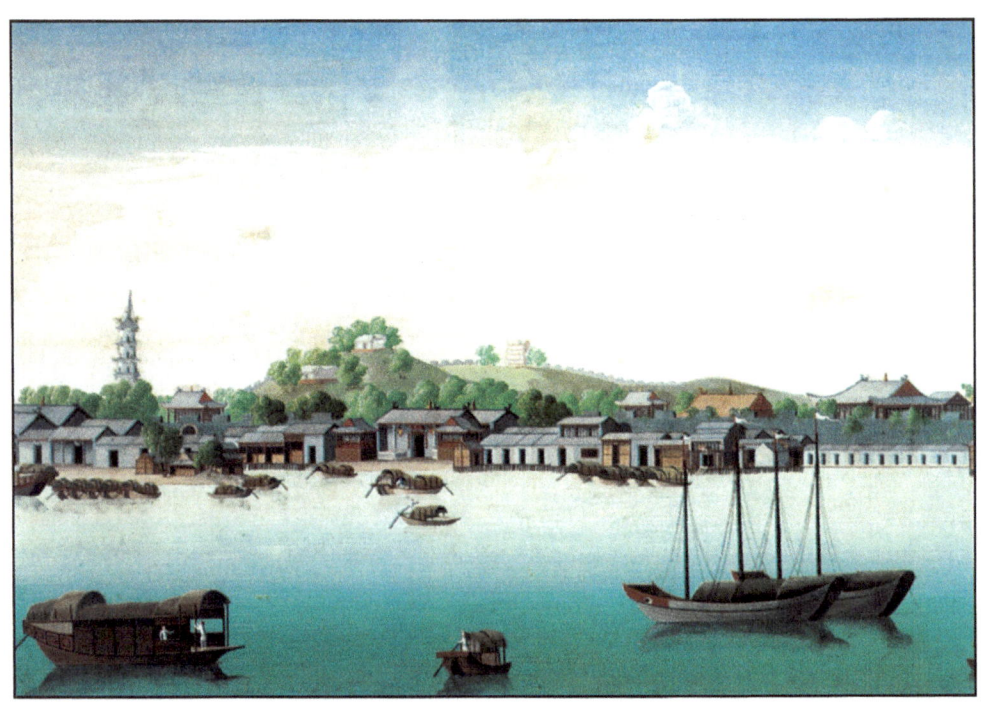

Foreign factories in Guangzhou c.1795.

HISTORICAL PERSPECTIVES

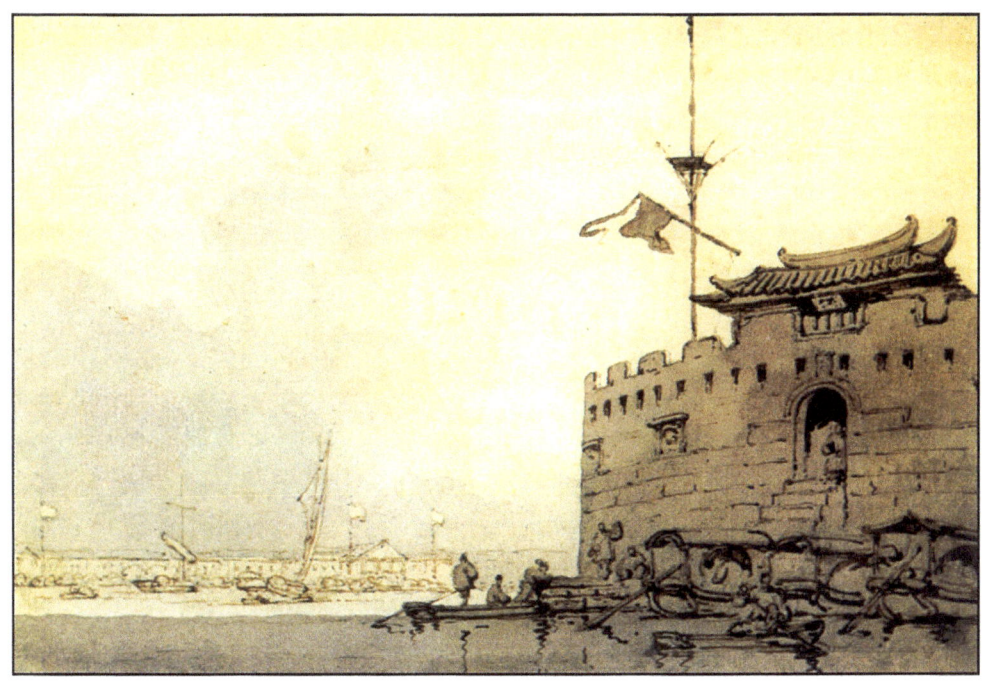

Dutch fort with Guangzhou in the background. G. Chinnery c. 1832.

The Portuguese first discovered the sea route linking Europe to South China in the 16th century[1]. Since then, trade between China and both Europe and the USA has flourished. By the middle of the eighteenth century, trade between Britain and the port of Canton (Guangzhou) was particularly active. The protectionist policy of the Chinese Government ensured that tea and silk were traded for only silver and gold. In an attempt to correct this imbalance, the British and Americans began to transport opium from Bengal to the Pearl River estuary and up to Canton. Thousands of the inhabitants of South China became addicted and the opium trade flourished. In 1838, the Emperor Daoguang at the Court of Peking was alarmed at the growing numbers of addicts and decided to crush the trade. He appointed Lin Zexu as Special Imperial Commissioner for the Suppression of the Opium Trade, who was dispatched to Guangdong, the southernmost province of China, adjacent to Hong Kong. In 1839, Lin ordered the seizure of all opium stocks which were confiscated and destroyed by mixing with lime in specially-constructed open pits, many of which survive intact today. Many foreign merchants were imprisoned for short periods.

In November 1839, the first battle of Chuen Pei occurred after High Commissioner Lin ordered the destruction of the English merchant ships by the Chinese military fleet. The Royal Navy attacked the Chinese fleet of war-junks and fire-rafts inflicting severe damage and the Chinese fleet subsequently withdrew. When the news of these events reached the British Parliament, a further seventeen Royal Navy warships were sent to the area in June 1840 and found safe anchorage in Hong Kong harbour. In the second battle of Chuen Pei, the Royal Navy assaulted the Chinese batteries at Tai Kok and Sha Kok which were the outer defences of the Bogue channel. The military operation was successful and the possession of Hong Kong was secured by treaty on January 30th 1841[2]. By April, the first buildings had been erected and the British administration of Hong Kong begun. Among the first buildings to be erected were the naval and military hospitals which were constructed from wooden frames and were quick and easy to erect. The reason why the building of hospitals was of importance was because the naval battles inflicted casualties and there was no appropriate place where they could be cared for.

Unfortunately, these early buildings were blown down in the typhoon of July 22nd 1841; "the over-crowded and badly built hospitals were all levelled to the ground and their fragments whirled through the air"[3]. All subsequent buildings were designed to withstand tropical storms. The core buildings of the Ruttonjee Sanatorium were ample proof of this. Despite an exposed location and numerous typhoons, the original structure stood intact for nearly 150 years and even survived the devastating typhoon of 1874.

After the arrival of a second Royal Navy fleet in 1842, there was a blockade of the Grand Canal outside Nanking (Nanjing). Subsequently, the Treaty of Nanking was signed in August 1842 which guaranteed free trade for the British in China. The development of Hong Kong as a port and trading centre for China was assured.

MEDICINE IN THE SOUTH CHINA REGION

The health problems in South China at that time were formidable, and Hong Kong soon earned the reputation as a white man's grave[4]. Conditions at the time are detailed in Admiralty records. For example, an account of January 1841 reads: "Sickness had already begun to prevail among our troops before they had reached Hong Kong. The eight days exposure which they had endured on the heights of Canton sowed the seeds of ague and dysentery which proved far more formidable enemies than any troops the Chinese could bring against us. After the lapse of a few days, and when the excitement of active operations on shore and the cheering influence of hope and novelty had subsided, the sickness spread amongst the men with alarming rapidity, so that at length, out of our small force, no less than 1100 men were upon the sick list at Hong Kong. Part of this alarming state of things must be attributed certainly to the pernicious influence of the atmosphere of Hong Kong itself at that season of the year. But every allowance must be made for the exposure which the men had undergone at Canton, and for the susceptibility of constitution produced by long confinement aboard ship. The germs of disease were planted in their bodies before the men returned to the harbour of Hong Kong, and therefore an undue stress was laid upon the unhealthiness of Hong Kong itself"[3].

In April 1841, the first ever Naval Court of Inquiry held in Hong Kong was convened to investigate the high death rate of sailors. It is likely that many of these deaths were due to malaria, known locally as Hong Kong fever[2]. However the fevers were not attributed at that time to the Anopheles mosquito, but to unhealthy vapours seeping through cracks in the earth. Consequently, most sailors were encouraged to stay on their ships and they remained relatively healthy if they did so. This was probably not due to clean air, but because the ships were out of flying range of the land-based mosquito. In 1843, when fever killed 24% of all the troops and 10% of all European civilians between May and October, the entire European garrison was moved out of barracks and onto the ships[4]. General d'Aguilar, the first Commander of British forces, remarked in 1845 on the state of health of his troops: "To have 700 effective men, it is necessary to maintain 1400"[3].

In those early days, sailors were discouraged from going ashore for fear of breathing the unhealthy air. The first hospitals in the region were established by the Portuguese in Macau as early as 1557[1]. However, Western medicine in China did not become active until 1838 with the founding of the China Medical Missionary Society which subsequently opened a hospital in Hong Kong in 1843[5].

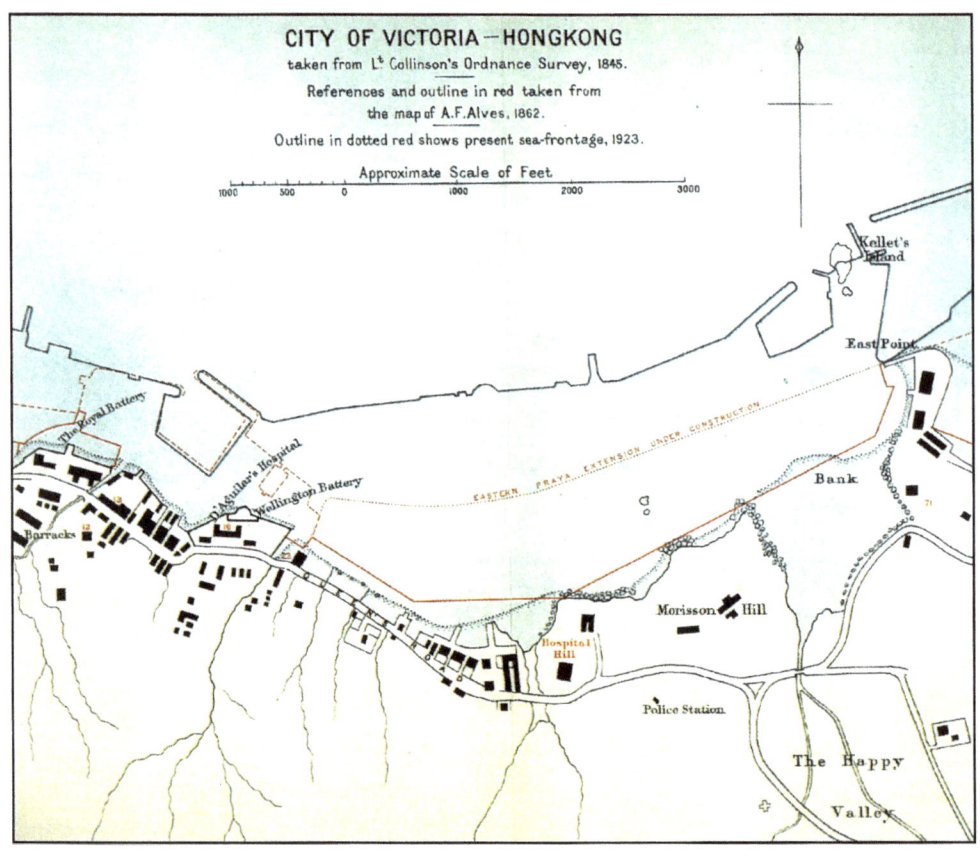

Map of Wanchai showing the Seamen's Hospital on Hospital Hill.

THE SEAMEN'S HOSPITAL 1843-1873

The original buildings of the Ruttonjee Sanatorium were first constructed as the Seamen's Hospital in 1842. The hospital was opened in 1843 and subsequently became the Royal Naval Hospital from 1873-1942. The idea of building the Seamen's Hospital was suggested by Mr. Heerjeebhoy Rustomjee (no relation to Ruttonjee), a Parsee merchant, who in 1841 offered money for the purpose of building the hospital. In the Hong Kong Gazette of July 15th 1841, there is a letter from Mr. Rustomjee to Dr. Alexander Anderson who at the time was Acting Surgeon to the British Superintendent of Trade. The donation was $12,000 for the building of a hospital to be used by foreign seamen, and the money was placed in the hands of Jardine Matheson and Co.

A committee comprising Messrs. Anderson, Matheson and Morrison was appointed to oversee the financing of the project but apparently there was a problem in securing payment from Mr. Rustomjee. Indeed, Mr. Rustomjee may have subsequently gone bankrupt. Eventually, Jardine Matheson and Co. had to find the funds to build the hospital. In addition to the funds made available by Jardines, there was a public subscription of $6000. The then Governor, Sir Henry Pottinger, allocated a site for the building of the hospital in February 1842, known as Inland Lot 86. The site was a hill overlooking Wanchai Gap, while the other three sides faced the sea as a bluff peninsula. The original plan was for a hospital of 50 beds and one residence for the hospital doctor. At that time, the area known as Wanchai was a fashionable district with large houses, well kept lawns and a waterfront promenade.

The hill on which the hospital was built marked the eastern end of the seafront promenade. A jetty and gate at the bottom of the hospital hill allowed patients to be unloaded from small boats and taken directly to the hospital wards. The original gate and arch still stand today and now open onto the busy market in Wanchai Road. An anchor motif is visible on one stone block, denoting the hospital's maritime association. The hospital was opened in August 1843, and the first superintendent was Dr. Peter Young, who founded the Hong Kong Dispensary now known as Watson's the chemist, and who was formerly the surgeon on the ship HMS Nemesis. Dr. Young gave his services free to the Seamen's Hospital, as did many of his successors. Subsequently, he was appointed Colonial Surgeon in 1846 following the death of Dr. Francis Dill.

He was an active member of the China Medico-Chirurgical Society which was founded on May 13th 1845, and he served as Treasurer for a short time.

In 1847, Dr. Young was one of the office-bearers of the China Medico-Chirurgical Society, which later became incorporated into the China Branch of the Royal Asiatic Society. The first President of the China Medico-Chirurgical Society was Dr. Tucker, a Ship's Surgeon on HMS Minden which had arrived in Hong Kong in June 1843. At the inaugural meeting, Tucker presented a synopsis of the first 1000 patients sent to HMS Minden for treatment. The most common ailment was dysentery (359 cases), followed by remittent fever (165 cases - probably malaria). The overall mortality was 31.5%. Dr. Tucker died aboard the Minden on September 10th 1845, while still holding the office of President. The Society subsequently developed into the Hong Kong Branch of the Royal Asiatic Society, most of whose founder members were medical practitioners[6].

In a letter written by Dr. Alexander Anderson to the Governor, Sir Henry Pottinger, on November 25th 1843, the details of the expenditure of the Rustomjee donation are recorded. The sum of $8500 had already been spent on erecting the building and the remaining $3500 would be needed for completion. The costs of admission to the Seamen's Hospital were defrayed by charges to the individual ships concerned. British subjects were also granted admission to the hospital, and the costs of these patients were met by the Government, who supported patients from the police and other Government departments. Reference is made in Dr. Anderson's letter to the situation of the hospital on top of the hill as "one well adapted for the purpose, being lofty and airy, and as far as can be judged from the health of the patients admitted there during the months when the greatest amount of sickness has prevailed upon the island since 1st August when the institution was opened - the locality is a healthy one"[7]. In the letter, Dr. Anderson requested a further $12,000 to expand the hospital and to build a house for a resident surgeon, which would enable him to give "the necessary medical attention".

In the final paragraph of the letter, Dr. Anderson pointed out that there were three British subjects in the hospital who were non-seamen, two of whom were being paid for privately and one "after the charity of the institution"[7]. The Governor, Sir Henry Pottinger, looked favourably on the activities of the

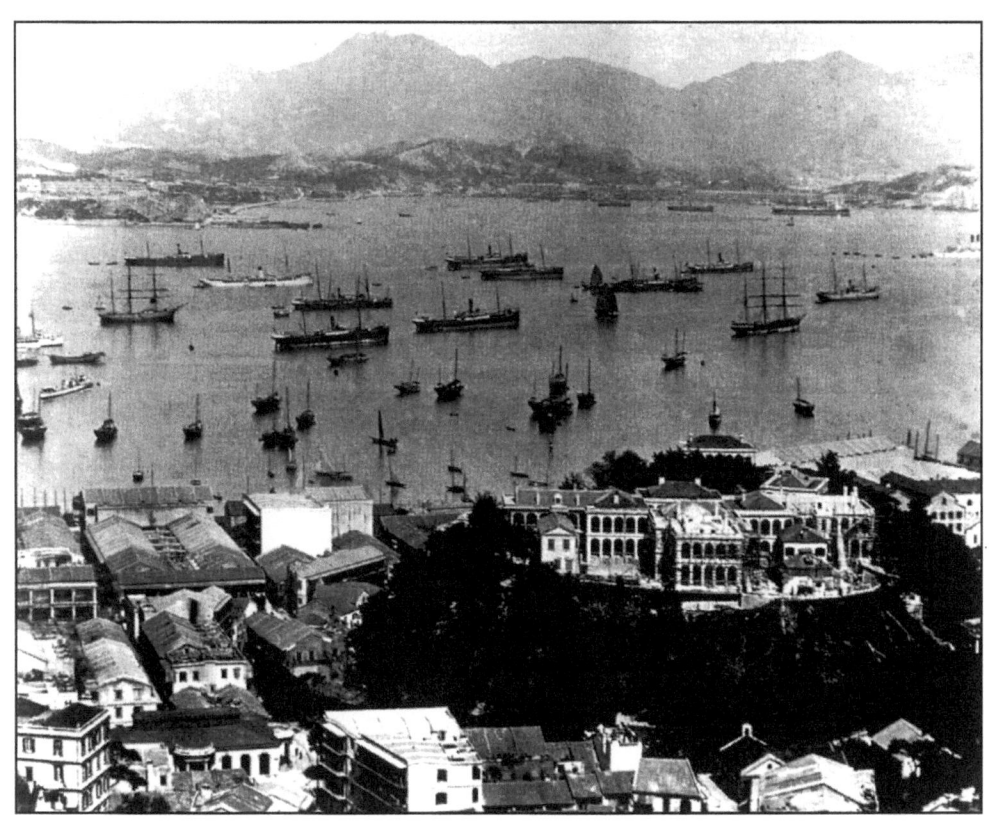

The Seamen's Hospital under renovation and reconstruction in 1873.

hospital and on November 28th 1843 wrote to Lord Stanley, Secretary of State for the Colonies, requesting additional funds (Appendix A). Funds were approved for the further extension of the hospital buildings, and a doctor's residence was erected. Dr. Young was appointed Colonial Surgeon on October 1st 1846, but how long he spent at the Seamen's Hospital is unclear. Also in that year, attempts were made by the next Governor, Sir John Davis, to dispel the myth that Hong Kong was an unhealthy place (Appendix B). Dr. William Harland compiled the annual report for the hospital for the year 1848, when there had been 203 admissions and 30 deaths, a mortality rate of 14.77%[8]. This mortality rate was higher than 1847 (11.02%) yet lower than 1846 (21.14%)[9].

In 1848, Dr. Harland described excessive mortality from pneumonia and acute dysentery; however intermittent fever (almost certainly malaria) was the most prevalent sickness during that year. The report also states that many patients were stricken with intermittent fevers while in the hospital for other conditions. There is reference to one ward being particularly affected: "In the month of August, particularly in one of the wards exposed to the Southwest winds blowing down the gap opposite the hospital, every patient during the afternoon was seized with an ague, and had repeated attacks notwithstanding the use of quinine, until removal onto another ward not similarly exposed. After removal they quickly got well and no cases occurred at the time in any other ward, that being the one so exposed"[8].

In the Colonial Surgeon's report of 1849, Dr. Harland remarked on the high prevalence of venereal disease amongst merchant seamen. Syphilis, gonorrhoea, strictures and rheumatism comprised 29.28% of all cases admitted to the hospital. On the Royal Navy Flag Ship Hastings, 100 of a crew of 300 men were suffering from venereal infections. Dr. Harland commented: "Venereal disease presents itself in this place in a form of particular virulence and malignity, such as, I believe, is rarely witnessed"[9]. In the Colonial Surgeon's report of 1850, there were 202 admissions, embracing a great variety of diseases of which fevers, dysentery, rheumatism, pulmonary and syphilitic afflictions were the most common.

The proportion of deaths for that year was 13.3%, but no figures are available for the year 1851, as Dr. Harland was ill. Most records concerning notifications of syphilis in the Royal Navy were subsequently destroyed by white ants in 1858, and the debris was burnt to destroy the larvae[10]. Dr. Harland was also a member of the China Medico-Chirurgical Society to which he presented a paper on "The Chinese System of Human Anatomy and Physiology" in 1847. He died by drowning while boating near Lamma Island in 1858, aged 34 years. In his will, Dr. Harland bequeathed most of his possessions to his Chinese amah. His natural history collection was bequeathed to the Scarborough Philosophical Society in Yorkshire, England.

The hospital was clearly busy and served a useful purpose, but in the early 1860's financial difficulties arose. Jardine Matheson and Co. took over the administration and rebuilt most of the hospital. It was re-opened in May 1866 but continued to run at a loss and was closed in March 1873.

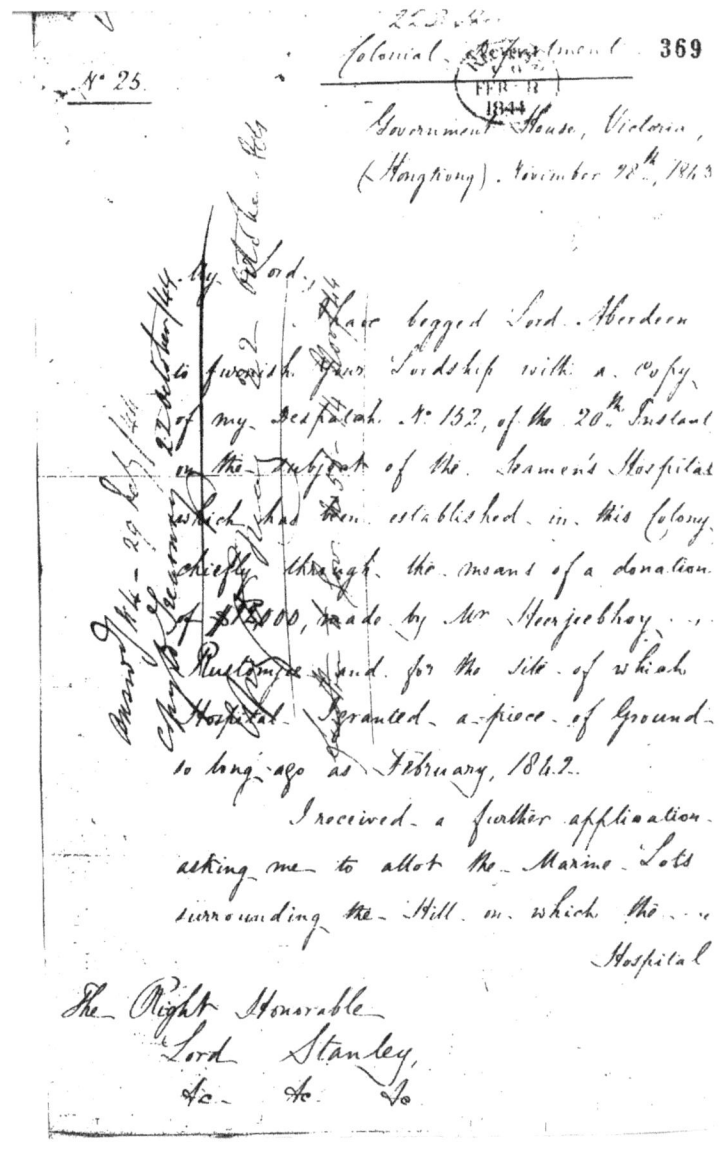

Letter from the Governor of Hong Kong, Sir Henry Pottinger, to Lord Stanley dated November 28th 1843, requesting further funds to increase the capacity of the Seamen's Hospital.

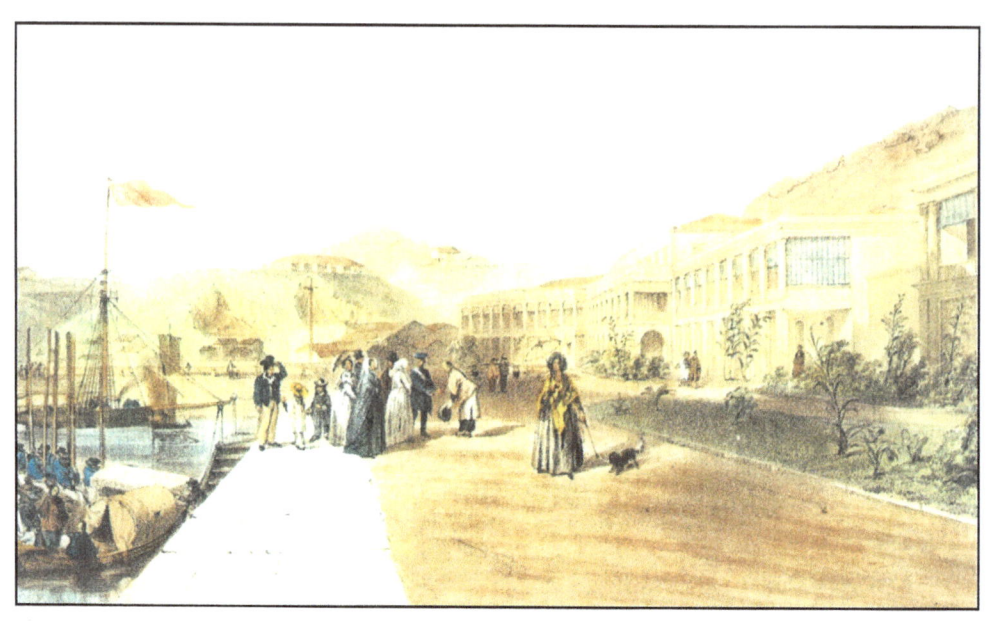

*Spring Gardens at Wanchai looking eastwards. M. Bruce 1846.
The Seamen's Hospital was situated on the hill at the end of the promenade.*

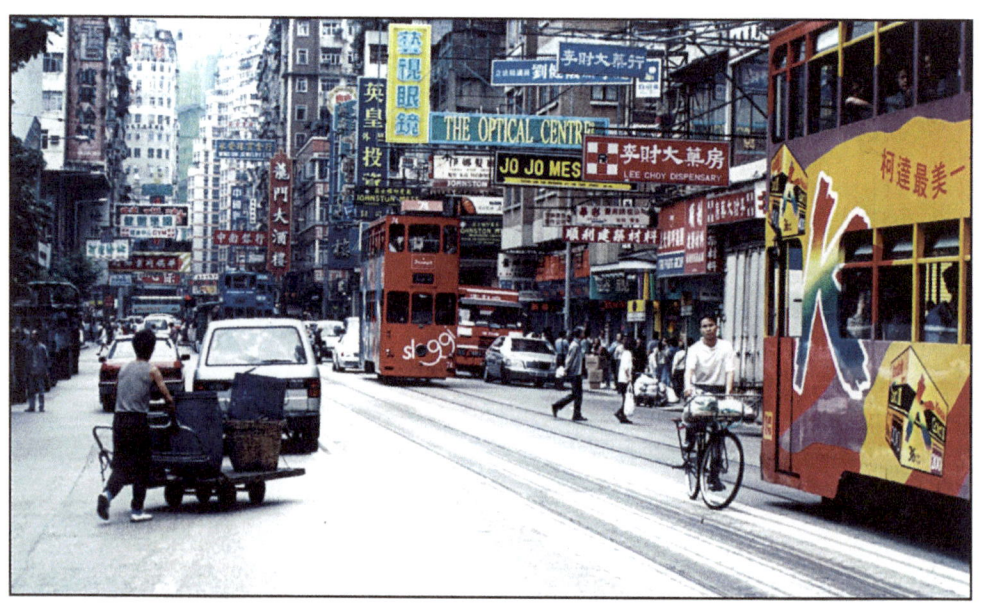

A view from approximately the same site in 1996, some 150 years later.

THE ROYAL NAVAL HOSPITAL 1873-1942

The Royal Navy had traditionally used hospital ships to care for their sick and wounded, but had been investigating the possibility of a shore-based hospital since 1865. The hospital ship in service in Hong Kong waters was HMS Melville, but she was thought no longer suitable to care for sick sailors. Conditions on the ship were generally poor, with cramped quarters, poor ventilation and light, and no room for patients to convalesce. Some sailors admitted to the ship subsequently contracted more lethal diseases than those for which they were admitted. There was therefore an urgent need to establish a shore-based facility in the colony.

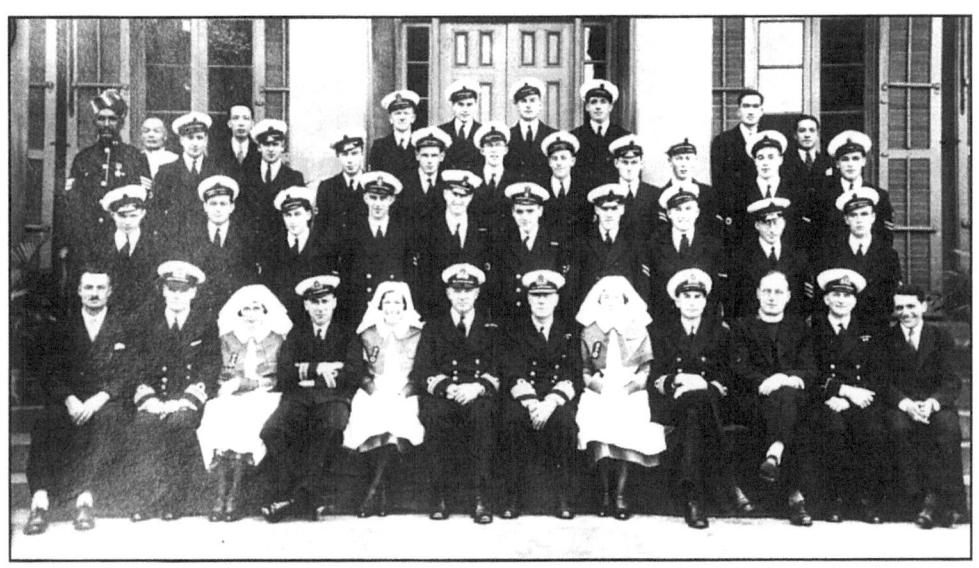

Staff of the Royal Naval Hospital, 1937-1940.

In 1873, the Seamen's Hospital was sold by Jardine Matheson and Co. to the Admiralty for the price of $35,000. HMS Melville was sold for $35,600 hence the Navy made a small profit in the transaction. The Admiralty undertook further reconstruction and some additional buildings were erected. A high wall was built around the entire site, parts of which remain intact today. Three lots of land adjacent to the hospital site were also purchased.

The Navy was delighted with their purchase and the site was named Mount Shadwell in honour of the Vice-Admiral of the China Station,

Charles A. Shadwell. The hospital was described as "perfect as it is possible to conceive. Four oblong blocks, two storeys, surrounded by verandahs and enclosing a central hollow quadrangle. The arrangement securing good light, ventilation, and space for exercise on the verandah. Lighted throughout with gas, and has an ample water supply from reservoirs on a neighbouring hill"[11]. At an elevation of 120 feet above sea level, the plot was open to the sea breeze and also the wind blowing down the valley below Wanchai Gap. The disadvantages of the site included mosquitoes and close proximity to a slaughterhouse for pigs "the squealing of which is a decided nuisance"[12]. The hospital opened with 10 beds for officers and 48 beds for seamen and marines, but was soon expanded to accommodate 106 patients. The hospital had an eventful history. In 1876 a large landslip occurred at the west end of the hospital site following heavy rain. There was considerable damage to property in the adjacent Wanchai Road. Local residents claimed damages from the Royal Navy as the landslip had originated on Admiralty property.

During the Franco-Chinese hostilities, a letter from the Foreign Office in April 1885 stated that the sick and wounded from either side could be admitted to the Royal Naval Hospital in Hong Kong without contravening any international rules. During the first year of the plague epidemic in 1894, which eventually claimed more than 2500 lives, naval surgeons participated in the care of plague victims at other hospitals.

By tradition, nursing staff in the Royal Navy were male. The possibility of employing female nurses was not realized until the 1890's, when efforts were made to obtain Nursing Sisters for the Royal Naval Hospital. There was no suitable accommodation in the hospital for female nurses and a separate house was built. The engagement of female nursing sisters had still not been achieved by 1897 and in a letter to Vice-Admiral Sir Alexander Buller from the Deputy Inspector of the hospital, the following paragraph appears: "The benefits of Nursing Sisters have been so amply proved and the comfort and help they give to patients is so generally recognized that the Royal Naval Hospital here must be considered as being behind the times without them.

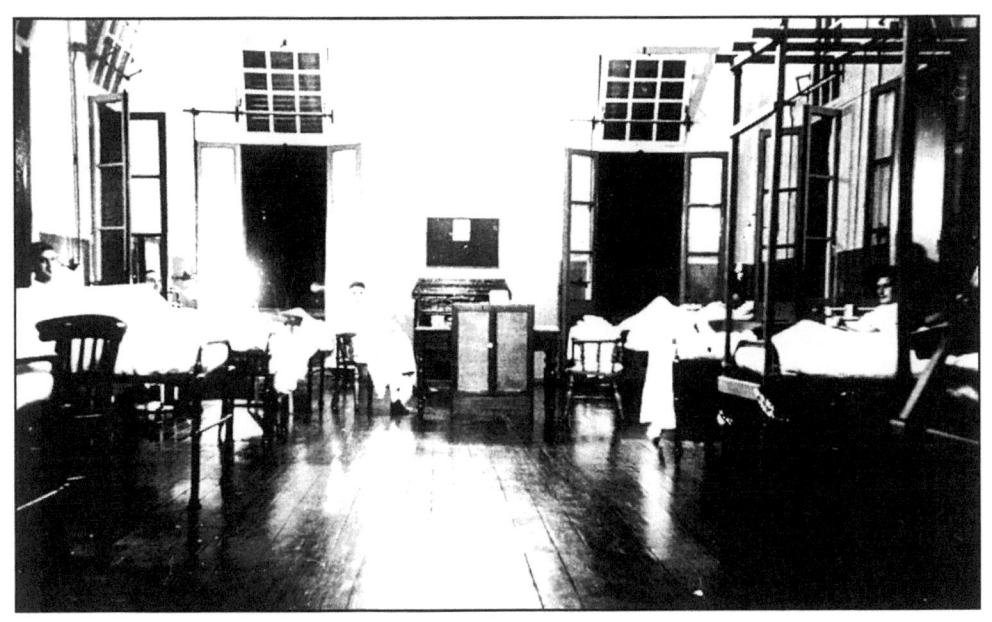

Ward and patients of the Royal Naval Hospital, 1938.

All the civilian hospitals in Hong Kong are well with them, and they stand the climate as well as other people"[3]. It was not until 1904 that Nursing Sisters were recruited from the Royal Navy Queen Alexandra's Nursing Service, members of which served in the hospital until 1942.

The Japanese assault on Hong Kong began on December 8th 1941 and many sailors were transferred back to their ships. The hospital was hit by many shells and on December 12th the staff quarters and operating theatres were badly hit. Gas, electricity and water supplies all failed. The roof was severely damaged and patients were evacuated to the ground floor. Numerous surgical operations were performed in the corridors by candlelight[13]. Although there was an extensive network of air-raid tunnels under the hospital, most staff were too busy to use them. Food and water were scarce, and at one point there was one bowl of water available to wash 12 patients. After the fall of Hong Kong on Christmas Day 1941, there was a further influx of casualties, stretching staff and facilities still further. On January 18th 1942, the Japanese ordered the evacuation of patients and staff, firstly to St. Albert's Convent and subsequently to the Military Hospital on Bowen Road, which still stands today.

At the end of the Second World War, the hospital was inspected by Surgeon-Commander D. F. Walsh on September 2nd 1945 after the re-occupation of Hong Kong. The hospital had suffered considerable structural damage in addition to being looted, and rehabilitation would have been a costly undertaking, practically amounting to rebuilding it. The roof was severely damaged, due to shelling by the Japanese. It was decided that it would be preferable to build a new hospital on another site, rather than spend a large sum on a hospital which was in such poor repair. Furthermore, Wanchai was no longer a fashionable residential district. With reclamation of the foreshore, the hospital became separated from the sea and was surrounded by a densely populated slum area "with all the attendant disadvantages of flies, smells, smoke and noise"[3].

The hospital was therefore abandoned by the Royal Navy, and the Royal Navy Medical Service subsequently occupied two floors of Queen Mary Hospital, and in 1947 moved to the War Memorial Nursing Home on Victoria Peak.

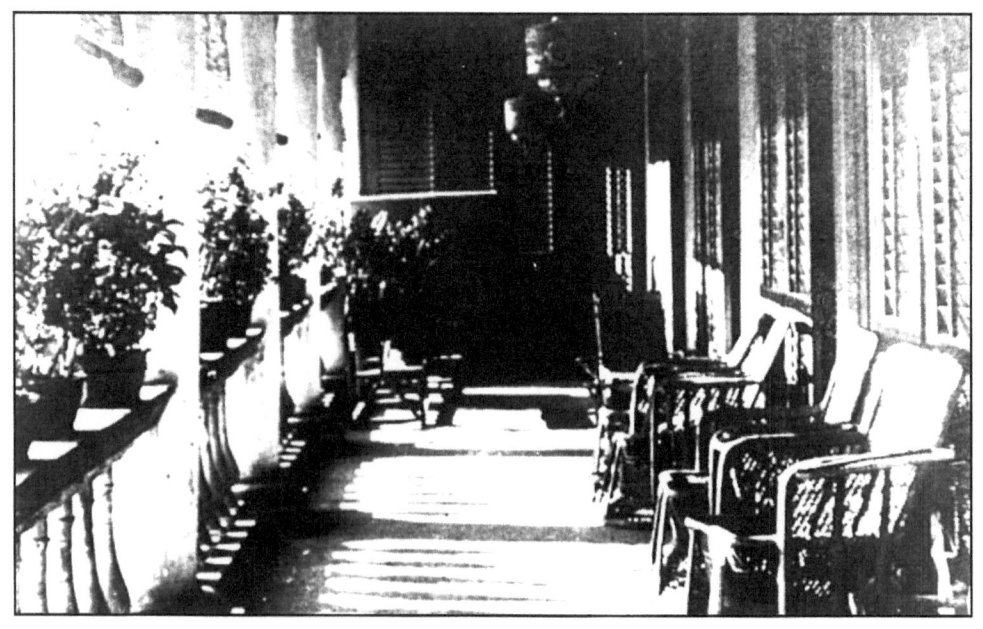

Verandah of the Royal Naval Hospital.

The Ruttonjee Family

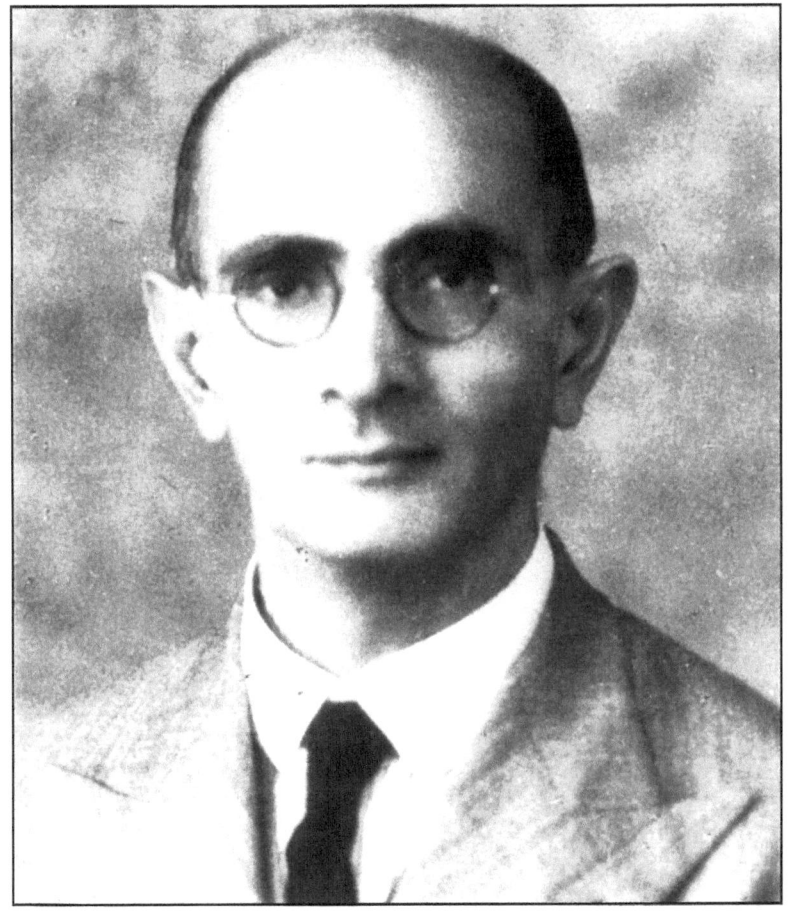

Mr. J. H. Ruttonjee, CBE, 1880-1960.

Mr. Jehangir Hormusjee Ruttonjee, CBE, was born in the small town of Bulsar in the Indian State of Gujarat. He was the only child of Mr. Hormusjee Ruttonjee and his wife Dina. Mr. Hormusjee Ruttonjee came to Hong Kong in 1880 and when he was well established here after a few years of hard work, he sent for his wife and 12-year-old son Jehangir, who landed in Hong Kong in 1892. The young boy entered the Victoria English School whose headmaster at that time was Mr. W. D. Braidwood. Mr. Jehangir Ruttonjee remained in Hong Kong and lived under 15 different governors. As a schoolboy, he received a prize from Sir William Robinson, Governor from 1891 to 1898.

In 1902, Mr. Jehangir Ruttonjee married Miss Banoo Master and from this marriage were born three daughters and a son, the well-known and respected Hon. Dhun Ruttonjee, CBE, who passed away in 1974.

During the Japanese occupation, many Hong Kong residents were grateful to Mr. Jehangir Ruttonjee for his aid for which he was twice arrested by the Japanese in 1942 and in 1944, together with his son Dhun. In 1944, after having been confined in prison on remand for 12 months, and subjected to the usual Japanese tortures, both father and son were sentenced to five years' imprisonment each, for pro-British activities. Liberation in 1945 was absolute to them both, in every sense of the word!

After the war, the Ruttonjee business was in a shambles and Mr. Jehangir Ruttonjee had to work very hard indeed to restore order to his business. After a few months, the old firm was once again functioning properly and he decided to take a holiday with his wife Banoo and grand-daughter, Miss Vera Ruttonjee Desai. The family visited Europe and the United States. In London in 1948, Mr. and Mrs. J. H. Ruttonjee, as well as their grand-daughter, had the great honour to meet King George VI and Queen Elizabeth during a Royal Garden Party at Buckingham Palace. They also met the Prime Minister, Mr. Clement Atlee. In Rome, the Ruttonjees were received in a private audience by His Holiness the Pope Pius XII, who greeted each of them in turn and inquired about conditions in Hong Kong.

THE FOUNDING OF THE HONG KONG ANTI-TUBERCULOSIS ASSOCIATION

It was in 1944 that Mr. Jehangir Ruttonjee had first conceived the idea of a sanatorium to help those suffering from tuberculosis and to combat this dreaded scourge which was then claiming many lives each year.

During the occupation of Hong Kong by the Japanese, Mr. Jehangir Ruttonjee's very dear eldest daughter, Tehmi, contracted tuberculosis and it was heartbreaking for him to watch her intense suffering and to realize that he was powerless to help her. Medicines were nowhere to be found in war-time Hong Kong and this led eventually to her death on June 3rd 1943.

As soon as the Pacific War ended, Mr. Jehangir Ruttonjee started his campaign against tuberculosis. He called on a number of close and influential friends and convinced them of the need to fight the disease. Together with dedicated citizens such as Sir S. N. Chau, Messrs. Ngan Shing Kwan, Shum Wai Yau, D. Benson, Lee Lu Cheung, and also together with his son, Dhun Ruttonjee, they formed the Hong Kong Anti-Tuberculosis Association, with himself as Chairman of the Board of Directors and with all these gentlemen as Directors. Dr. S. N. Chau was an ear, nose and throat surgeon who left medical practice in favour of banking and subsequently became Chairman of the Chinese Bank. He gave many years of public service and was a member of the Urban, Legislative and Executive Councils. Mr Benson, as Chief Manager of the Mercantile Bank, was another prominent member of the business community. Mr. Jehangir Ruttonjee made enquiries for a site which would be suitable to build a sanatorium that could be expanded later, if circumstances should so dictate. He eventually found the former Royal Naval Hospital in Wanchai Road, which was disused and in an extremely dilapidated condition due to the looting of fixtures during the war. He donated generously to the Association to the extent of $800,000 for the rehabilitation of the former Royal Naval Hospital site and for the building of the Ruttonjee Sanatorium thereon, and construction was fully completed in early 1949.

During the immediate post-war period, doctors, nurses, and all other hospital staff, as well as hospital equipment were extremely scarce. However, Mr. Jehangir Ruttonjee was not discouraged. He searched far and wide and was fortunate enough to contact the Columban Sisters in Ireland who were willing to undertake the management of the Sanatorium. An agreement was reached with Sisters of the

Order of Saint Columban to work as doctors and nurses in the Ruttonjee Sanatorium which became fully operational in February 1949. At the end of 1988, the Sisters finally withdrew from the services of the Hong Kong Tuberculosis, Chest and Heart Diseases Association.

Mr. Jehangir Ruttonjee made another generous donation of $300,000 to establish the Freni Memorial Convalescent Home in memory of his second daughter, Freni, who died of cancer in 1953. This was intended to relieve extreme over-crowding at the Sanatorium and to release 110 bed-spaces for tuberculosis patients. Convalescent male patients were in fact housed in the Freni Home at Mount Parish (Shiu Fai Terrace, reached via Stubbs Road) which is very near the Ruttonjee Sanatorium, until December 1991.

When Mr. Jehangir Ruttonjee passed away in February 1960 his son, the Hon. Dhun Ruttonjee, continued dedicating himself to the work of the Association. The Hon. Dhun Ruttonjee was a Director from the inception of the Association in 1948 and served actively on its sub-committees. He was a pioneer in the planning and formation of the 625-bed Grantham Hospital in Hong Kong, the foremost "Heart Hospital" in Southeast Asia. This hospital is also administered by the Association. He was elected Vice Chairman in June 1963 and Chairman in June 1964, and served in that capacity until his death in July 1974. The Hon. Dhun Ruttonjee was responsible not only for the long-term policy and expansion-plans of the Association, but also for the day-to-day administration. The result of his hard work, and that of the Association, was a significant reduction in the rates of both morbidity and mortality from tuberculosis in Hong Kong. He was well-known and recognized, both locally and internationally.

The connection between the Association and the Ruttonjee family did not end with the passing of the Hon. Dhun Ruttonjee in July 1974. Mr. R. M. Shroff, a grand nephew of Mr. Jehangir Ruttonjee joined the Board of Directors in March 1971 and was elected Vice Chairman in January 1975, and Chairman in March 1983. He is carrying on the fine traditions handed down by the late Mr. Jehangir Ruttonjee and the late Hon. Dhun Ruttonjee. Furthermore, Miss Vera Ruttonjee-Desai, the grand-daughter of the founder of the original Association, is on the Board of Directors of the Association.

THE RUTTONJEE SANATORIUM 1949-1991

At the end of World War II, tuberculosis was rampant in Hong Kong where it was the leading cause of death. In 1949, there were 7510 notifications of tuberculosis (a rate of 404 per 100,000 population) and 2611 deaths. The notification rates remained at this high level until 1962, before starting to decline significantly, but the proportion of patients dying from tuberculosis had started to decline rapidly from 1953. Under the chairmanship of Mr. J. H. Ruttonjee, the Hong Kong Anti-Tuberculosis Association joined with the government in the fight against the disease.

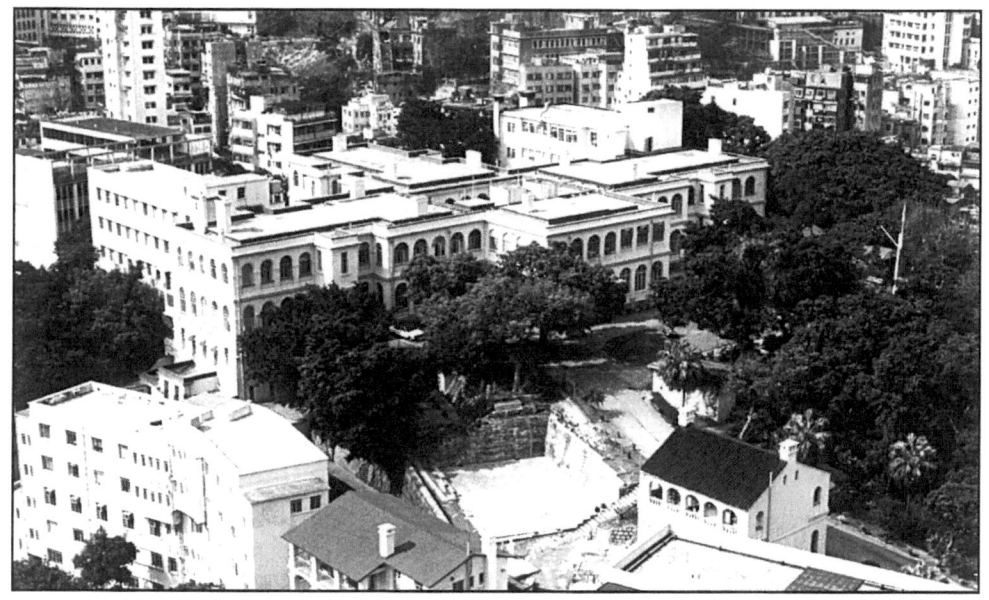

The view of the Ruttonjee Sanatorium from the Northeast. Over the years there has been extensive land reclamation and urban development around the site.

The Association felt that a religious order would be appropriate to administer the Sanatorium to provide continuous and dedicated service. Following the communist takeover in China in the late 1940's, many missionary orders had left the mainland and came to Hong Kong, either to be re-located to other parts of the world or to serve in the colony. At that time (1947) Mother M. Vianney, Superior General of the Columban Sisters, was in Hong Kong, having completed a visit to Sisters in China. The Columban Sisters were founded in Ireland in 1922 for missionary work in China. Though the first foundations were confined to China, later years brought expansion to the Philippines, Burma, Korea, South America and Pakistan.

In China, the Sisters opened and staffed hospitals and clinics in Hanyang, which is near Wuhan, and Nanchang in Jiangxi Province. Out-patient clinics were also operated to respond to emergency needs during epidemics of cholera, typhoid and dysentery. In Shanghai, the Sisters ran a school for children of Russian refugees.

Mother Vianney was asked if she would consider taking on the administration of the Sanatorium. In due course, the Columban Sisters agreed to administer the Sanatorium and in late 1947, Sisters Dolorosa and Catherine were released from the hospital in Hanyang, and came to Hong Kong to begin the work of refurbishing the Sanatorium. The old building was in an appalling state of disrepair and the two Sisters faced a formidable task. In the spring of 1948, Sisters Martin and de Chantal, both nurses, were withdrawn from Hanyang and sent to the Brompton Hospital in London, to gain experience in chest diseases.

Sister Mary Aquinas, a physician, was at this time also gaining experience at the Brompton. In early 1949, the staff members were Sisters Aquinas, Gerard, Martin, de Chantal, Francis Borgia and Dr. Mary Clifford. Miss Clare Mason and Miss Mary Dwyer (both nurses) also arrived from Ireland. Sister Aquinas and Dr. Clifford were the only medical staff. Three Columban Sisters also arrived from Shanghai; Sister Basil, a radiographer, Sister Anastasia, trained for office work, and Sister Bernadette, a nurse. Sister Clare, another nurse, arrived from Burma. On February 24th 1949, the Ruttonjee Sanatorium was officially opened by the Governor, Sir Alexander Grantham, with a bed occupancy for 60 patients. This number was soon increased to 214 as more staff and facilities were made available. In 1950, Sister M. Gabriel, a qualified doctor, joined the staff as did Sisters Martha, Aidan and Damien. Professor A. J. S. MacFadzean of the University of Hong Kong invited Sisters Aquinas and Gabriel in 1952 to lecture to the medical undergraduates from the University of Hong Kong, a task they performed for more than 30 years.

The hospital was recognized as a teaching hospital for graduates and undergraduates from the University of Hong Kong, and in the following years every medical graduate was taught at the Ruttonjee Sanatorium and quite a number served on the staff. In October 1952, the Sanatorium was honoured by an official visit from HRH Princess Marina, the Duchess of Kent.

In 1953, BCG vaccination was offered to the people of Hong Kong for the first time, and proved to be very popular. Funds were donated by the Jockey Club to build a new wing of the Ruttonjee Sanatorium in 1953 which was officially opened by Sir Arthur Morse, the Chairman of the Jockey Club. This extension provided three new airy wards with extra bed capacity for 66 patients.

In December 1953, the first Central Sterile Supply Department in Hong Kong was opened at the Sanatorium, and the operating theatre was functioning by 1954. Dr. Kenneth Hui, Senior Lecturer at the Department of Surgery, the University of Hong Kong, performed the first thoracoplasty in the Sanatorium on March 20th 1954, and contributed a number of publications[14,15]. Dr. A. R. Hodgson, Senior Lecturer in Orthopaedics, undertook surgery for tuberculosis of the spine. The first anterior spinal fusion was performed on April 10th 1954, a procedure which subsequently became known as "the Hong Kong Operation"[16]. Both surgeons provided free services to the Sanatorium for many years.

My own relatively brief sojourn at the Sanatorium was the six-year period from 1984-1989. As a physician newly arrived from England where tuberculosis is relatively rare, seeing more than 300 patients under one roof with the disease was a dramatic change. We witnessed the most severe presentations of the disease and saw tuberculosis in all of its protean forms. The overwhelming majority of patients recovered and this was very gratifying, but we also saw the ravages and horror of tuberculosis. Trying to manage patients coughing volumes of fresh blood was a challenge, and we were regularly rendered helpless by the rapid demise of emaciated patients with extensive disease who would survive only days, or sometimes only hours, after admission. Thankfully, the atmosphere was very supportive and was rather like working in a family house with a large number of guests, rather than working in a hospital. The professionalism, energy, dedication and humour of the Sisters was infectious. They were also highly skilled administrators and had many friends. A number of university specialists and private practitioners would visit patients in the wards on an entirely honorary basis. Professor Arthur Yau, Dr. Harry Fang and Dr. Louis Hsu of the University of Hong Kong, would visit regularly and their orthopaedic expertise was particularly valued and appreciated.

Funds for the first physiotherapist were allocated in 1969 and Mrs. Susan Finzel was employed on a part-time basis. Mrs. Susan Finzel remained with the Ruttonjee Sanatorium, apart from a break in the mid seventies, until 1992. An increase in the size of the establishment was hampered by recruitment difficulties which were overcome in 1971 by the decision to sponsor a student on the new physiotherapy course at Hong Kong Polytechnic. This required a commitment to work for the Sponsor for three post-graduate years. A second student was sponsored in 1978, to maintain the establishment at two staff.

The case load was initially physiotherapy for assorted acute and chronic chest conditions, including pre- and post-surgery, which was then being performed in the Sanatorium. Treatment was also given for various physical disabilities resulting from tuberculous meningitis, and also rehabilitation for post-orthopaedic surgery, including tuberculosis of the spine. In 1992, geriatric wards were established and a full range of physiotherapy for multi-pathological conditions for the elderly were added to the workload.

Sister Mary Greaney joined the nursing staff in 1971 and became Matron in 1982. Sister Nancy Kwok was appointed Matron in 1988 on the retirement of Sister Mary Greaney.

The number of patients (up to 350) for the relatively small staff meant hard work and long hours but it was a pleasure to be there in such a unique environment. The Sanatorium itself was an impressive structure with spacious wards and verandahs, high ceilings and a broad, open vista catching any breeze that might be blowing. The site was surrounded by riotous vegetation and banyan trees, many of them rare species. However, the condition of the buildings deteriorated, and with the development of the new hospital the old structure was demolished in March 1992, nearly 150 years after the first buildings were erected on the site.

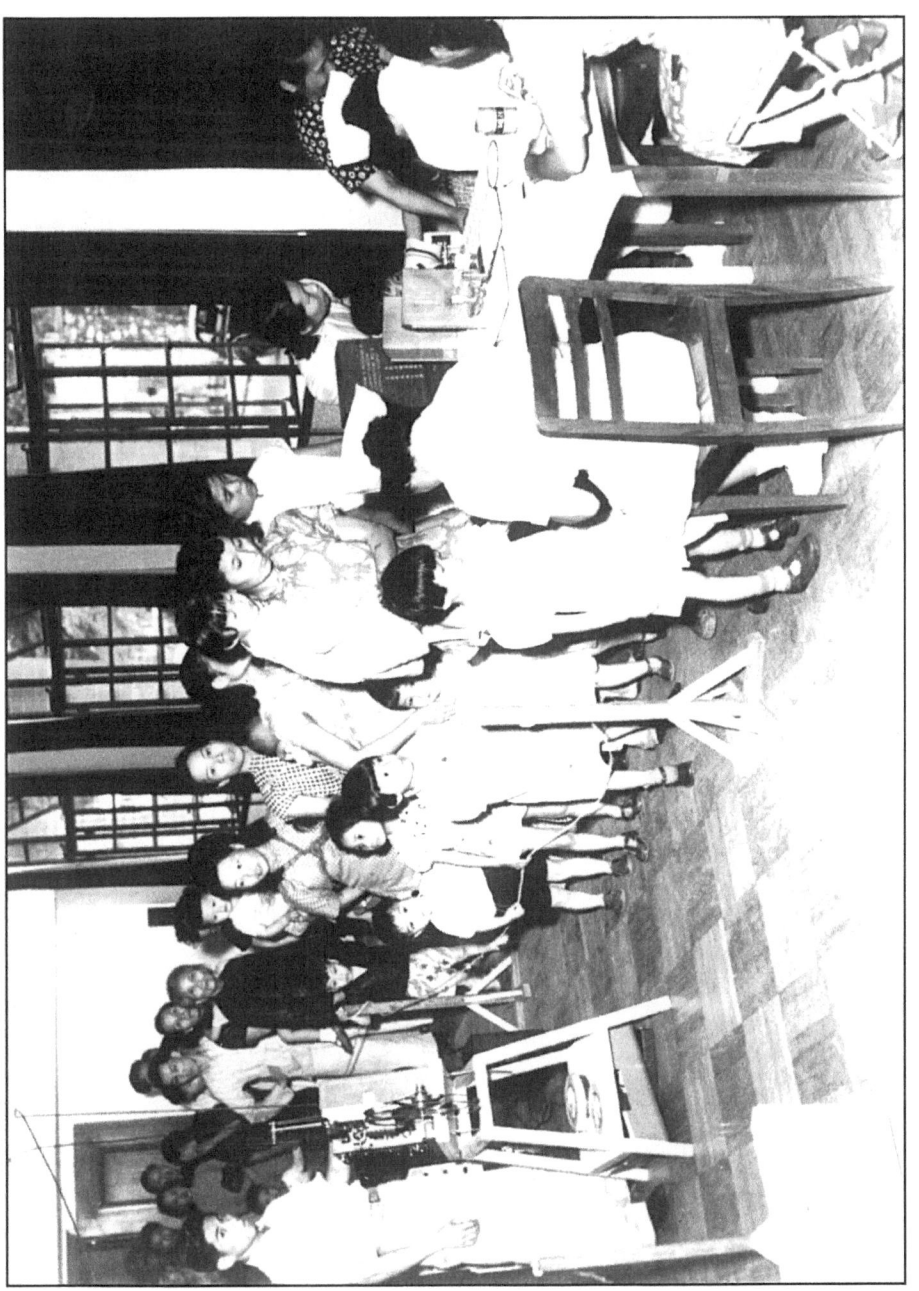

Children receiving BCG vaccination in 1953.

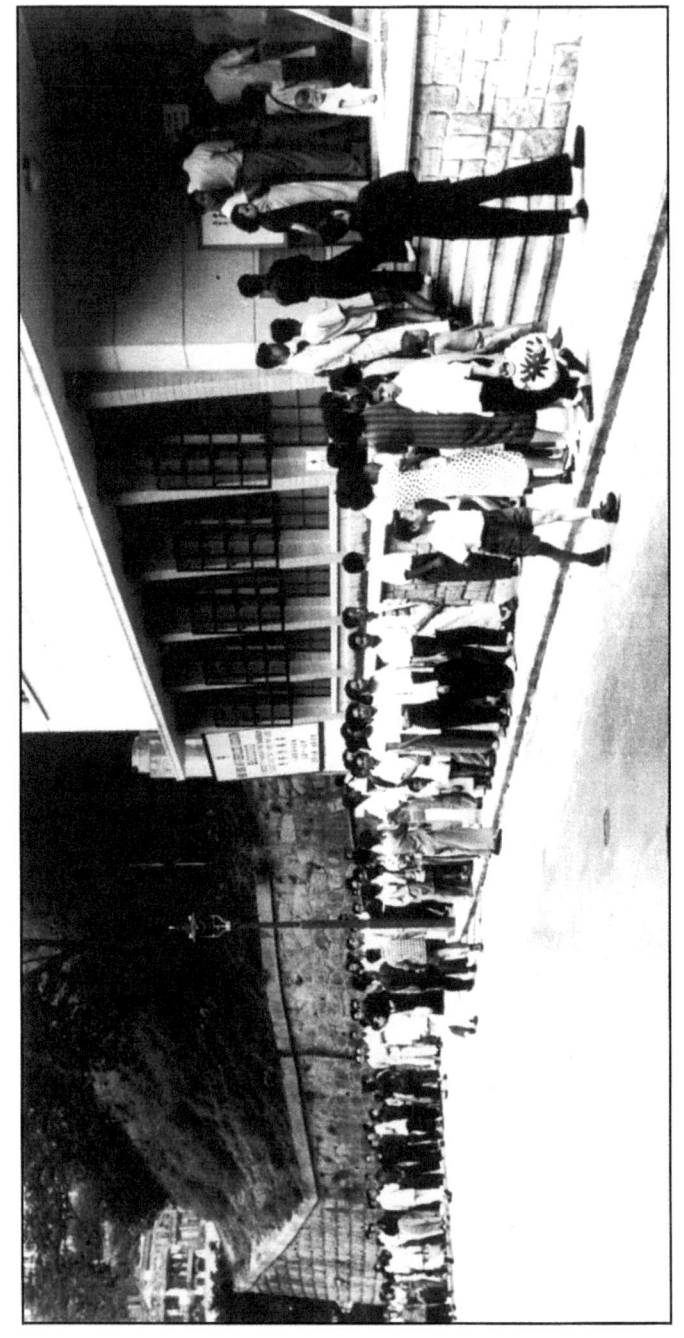

The queue for BCG vaccination outside the Ruttonjee Sanatorium in 1953.

Contributions to the Fight Against Tuberculosis

Statistics published by the Hong Kong Government Chest Service reveal that tuberculosis has been a significant cause of morbidity and mortality in the territory since the turn of the century. However it is likely that the disease has seriously afflicted earlier generations. In the year 1900, a total of 845 people died from tuberculosis, a mortality rate of 200 per 100,000 of the population. In 1920, the death toll was 2082, a rate of 320 per 100,000.

In the absence of effective treatment, the death toll from tuberculosis in the pre-war years was significant. In 1939, the last year that statistics are available prior to the Japanese occupation of Hong Kong, the disease claimed 4443 persons, a rate of 250 per 100,000.

While the situation in the pre-war years was unhealthy, the Second World War and the Japanese occupation made the situation much worse. With social distruption, poor nutrition and severe overcrowding, it is likely that tuberculosis claimed many lives during the war years although no figures are available. In the post-war period tuberculosis was the leading cause of death in the territory and control of the disease was made more difficult by the arrival of thousands of refugees from China. In 1946, there were 2801 notifications of new tuberculosis patients, and 1752 deaths. In that year the average age of death from tuberculosis was just 25 years, demonstrating that a significant number of those who died were children and young adults. During the period 1946 to 1955, there was a steep increase in the numbers of patients with tuberculosis, in 1955 alone there were more than 14,000 new notifications and 2800 deaths.

Fortunately, in the late 1940's and early 1950's real progress in the development of anti-tuberculosis medication had been achieved and streptomycin, isoniazid and para-aminosalicylic acid (PAS) quickly became available in Hong Kong. Following the alarming increase in tuberculosis in the post-war years a comprehensive programme was developed to combat the problem which included measures initiated both by the Government and the Anti-Tuberculosis Association. These included the building of new hospitals, the introduction of BCG vaccination, and the establishment of outpatient clinics especially for the treatment of tuberculosis. Many of the Government's efforts were planned and co-ordinated by Dr. K. C. Yeo and Dr. D. J. M. Mackenzie.

The importance of compliance with therapy as a key factor in success was realised by Dr. Alan Moodie, a tuberculosis specialist who introduced the concept of supervised treatment whereby the patient is directly observed taking their medication so as to avoid non-compliance. This system was established in the early 1950's in Hong Kong. Interestingly, this method of supervising treatment has recently been recommended in the USA, forty years later than the initiative taken in Hong Kong.

Following these measures the epidemic gradually came under control and by 1970 the number of new patients had declined to 10,077 (1436 deaths) and the general downward trend has continued ever since. Of particular interest is the rapid decline in mortality from tuberculosis, due mostly to the effectiveness of anti-tuberculosis treatment. Whereas in 1900, the mortality rate from tuberculosis was 200 per 100,000, the rate had fallen to 6.7 per 100,000 by 1994. This is a remarkable achievement, however, it should be remembered that tuberculosis has claimed nearly 150,000 lives in Hong Kong since 1900, and continues to claim nearly 400 citizens each year.

Over the past 40 years, the incidence of tuberculosis in Hong Kong has declined due to many factors, including the rise in the standard of living bringing better housing and nutrition, and the BCG vaccination programme which currently has a coverage of over 99% of newborns in Hong Kong. The BCG programme was particularly important in reducing severe forms of childhood tuberculosis and associated mortality from the disease. Perhaps the most important contribution was the availability of effective anti-tuberculosis treatment which was given free of charge on a fully supervised in-patient or out-patient basis. While the Ruttonjee Sanatorium always played a key role in the hospital management of tuberculosis, a significant contribution was also made in research studies of two new drugs, rifampicin and pyrazinamide. The availability of these new agents meant that the duration of treatment could be shortened considerably to six months, in contrast to the then standard 18-month drug regimens.

The Association and the Ruttonjee Sanatorium, in conjunction with the Government Chest Service headed initially by Dr. G. Allan and subsequently by Dr. S. L. Chan, collaborated with the British Medical Research Council (MRC) in studies relating to anti-tuberculosis treatment schedules for use in Hong Kong and elsewhere. Professor Wallace Fox as the Director of the MRC Tuberculosis and Chest Diseases Unit, and Professor Denny Mitchison of the MRC Unit for Laboratory Studies in Tuberculosis, played key roles in this research programme over a 25-year period. Their vision, leadership and hard work enabled the development of effective short-course chemotherapy for tuberculosis patients.

The many publications that emerged from the MRC/Hong Kong Government Chest Service collaboration, together with other MRC projects, had an enormous impact on the treatment of tuberculosis worldwide. These included definitive controlled clinical studies to identify optimum chemotherapy regimens for sputum smear-positive[17-22] and smear-negative[23,24] pulmonary tuberculosis, and important contributions concerning re-treatment[25], bacteriology[26], and adverse reactions to therapy[27-30]. Recent studies have further shortened the duration of the initial intensive phase of treatment[31], thereby reducing costs and improving tolerability. Of the many significant advances in the treatment of tuberculosis elucidated in Hong Kong, the practical advantages, efficacy and tolerability of supervised, intermittent treatment is outstanding[21,31], particularly as an aid to improving patient compliance[32].

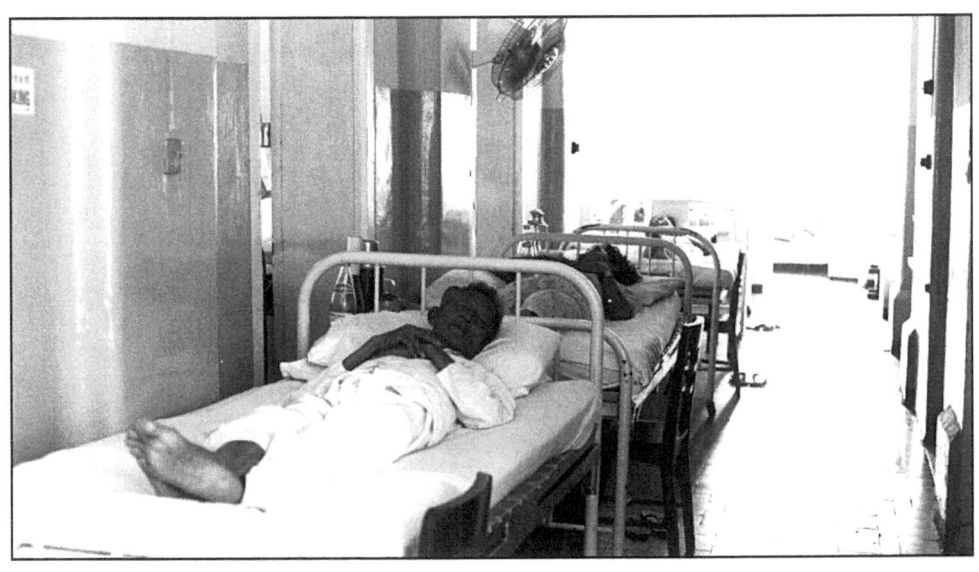

Patients with tuberculosis on the verandah of the Sanatorium.

The contribution of the Hong Kong Government Chest Service and the Ruttonjee Sanatorium to the treatment of tuberculosis is significant, and is probably Hong Kong's greatest contribution to medical research. A number of the treatment schedules and research findings are now standard clinical practice in many countries throughout the world, and have assumed a special importance as the incidence of tuberculosis is rising alarmingly in Africa, parts of Asia and the USA, secondary to the AIDS pandemic.

In 1975, Dr. G. H. Choa, then Director of Medical and Health Services, invited Professor Wallace Fox and Professor J. G. Scadding from the Brompton Hospital to visit Hong Kong to review the control and treatment of tuberculosis and to advise on future planning. With continued emphasis on outpatient chemotherapy and in view of the deteriorating physical state of the Ruttonjee Sanatorium, it was decided that a new hospital should be built to include more general medical and surgical facilities.

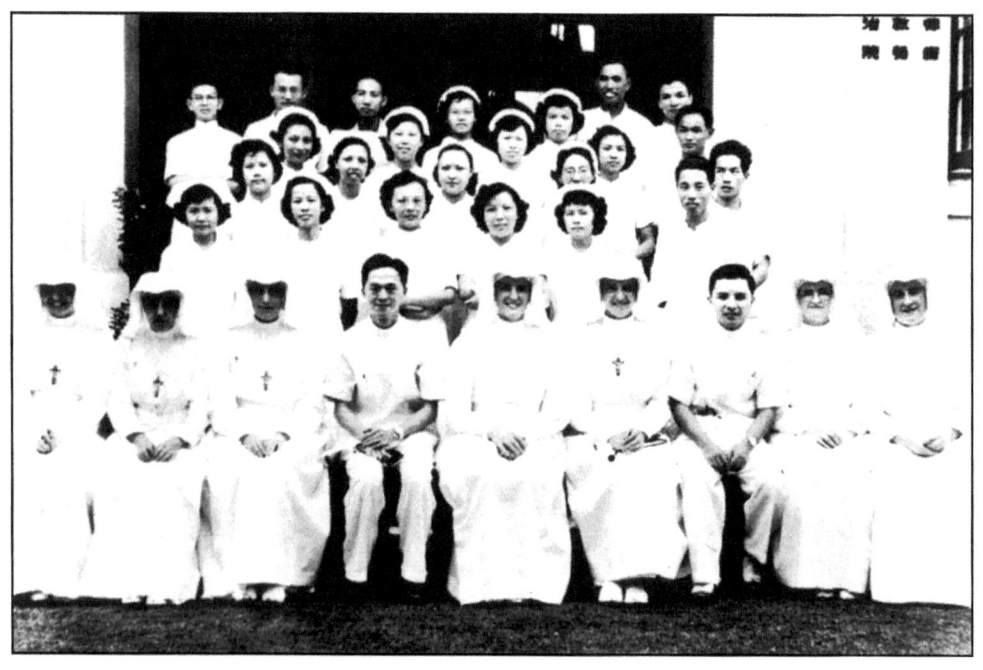

Staff of the Ruttonjee Sanatorium in 1952.

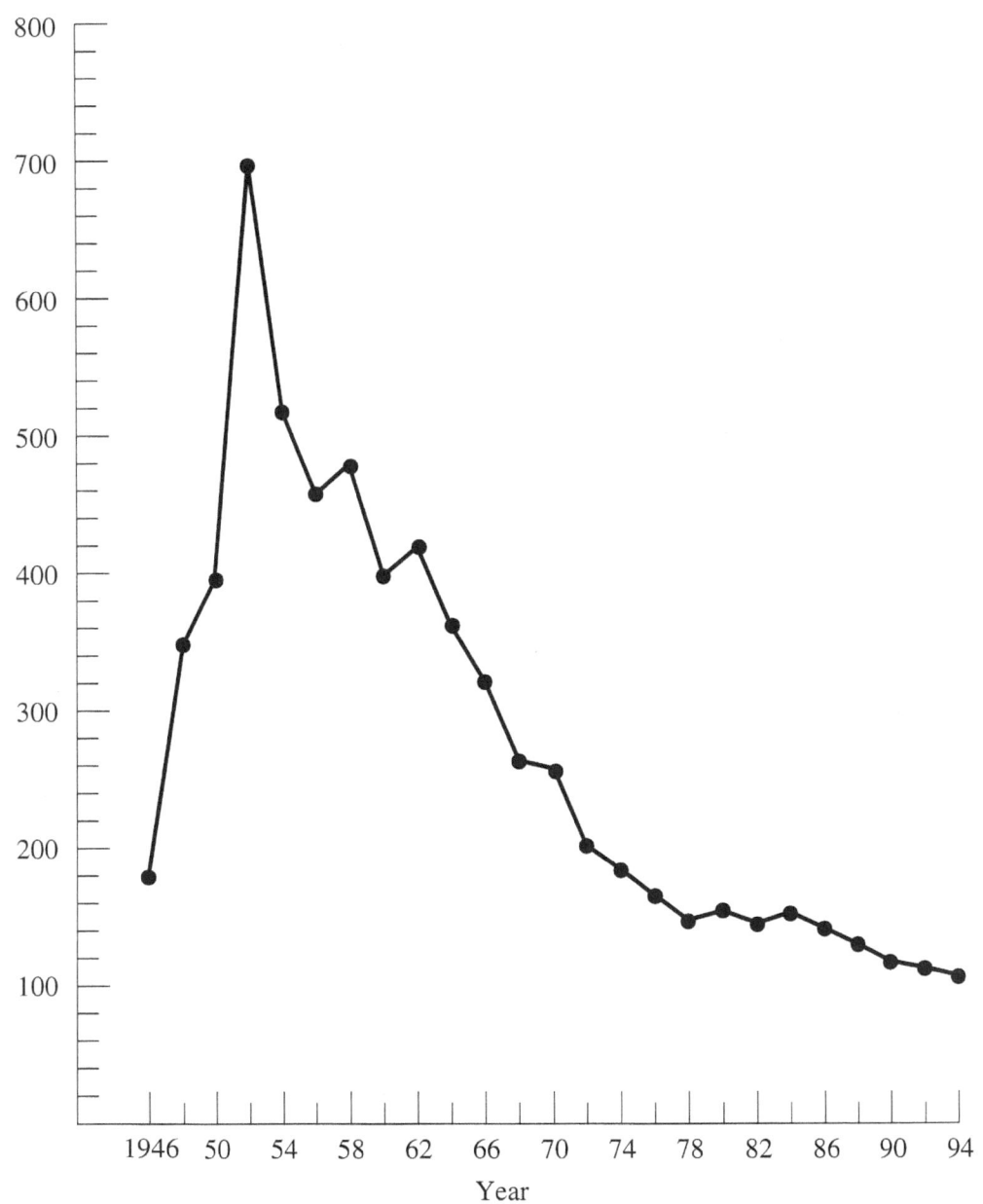

Notifications of tuberculosis in Hong Kong 1946-1994.
(Rate per 100,000 population)

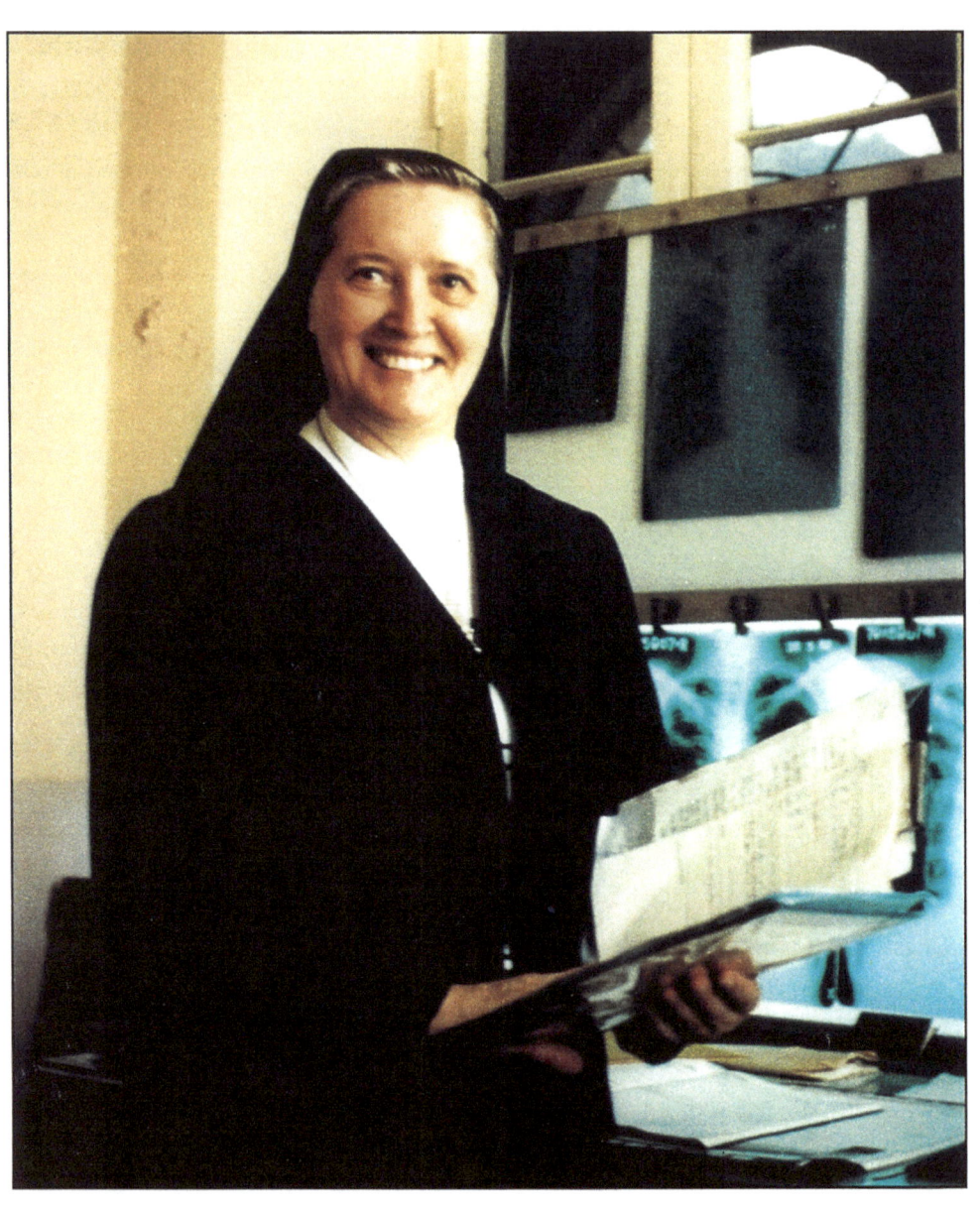

Sister Mary Aquinas, OBE, FRCP.
Medical Superintendent at Ruttonjee Sanatorium
1950-1985.

Sister Mary Aquinas

The Columban Sisters were under the leadership of the late Sister Mary Aquinas, OBE, FRCP, who was Medical Superintendent of the Ruttonjee Sanatorium for nearly 40 years. Sister Aquinas graduated in medicine from University College, Dublin, in 1947, having joined the Columban sisters in 1939. She was destined to work in China, but after Mao Zedong expelled the missionaries from China in 1949, she was posted to the Ruttonjee Sanatorium instead. For those of us who were privileged to know Sister Aquinas, words are hardly necessary. Her administrative and clinical skills, boundless energy and sense of humour are legendary. Internationally, she was sought after for the clarity of her teaching as well as for her wisdom in applying knowledge to developing countries, particularly in Asia. Her special research interests were drug resistance and re-treatment[33-37], and adverse reactions to anti-tuberculosis drugs[38-40]. Sister Aquinas also produced publications on the treatment and control of tuberculosis[41-45], BCG vaccination[46], and together with Professor Sir David Todd of the University of Hong Kong, a contribution to the Oxford Textbook of Medicine[47].

She was invited frequently by the World Health Organization and International Union Against Tuberculosis to participate in programmes to train doctors in Asia and Africa. In 1960, Sister Aquinas was the recipient of a Commonwealth Medal at the opening of the World Asthma Conference in Eastbourne. HRH Princess Marina presented the Sir Robert Philip Medal to Sister Aquinas for outstanding work in the field of tuberculosis in the Commonwealth. In 1978, the University of Hong Kong conferred on her the degree of Doctor of Social Sciences. In 1980, she was awarded the Order of the British Empire in recognition of her distinguished service in the fight against tuberculosis in Hong Kong, and was presented to Her Majesty Queen Elizabeth II at Buckingham Palace in the summer of 1985.

Sister Aquinas was keenly aware of the realities of working within a charitable organisation. One benefactor once donated an extravagant array of flowers to the hospital, about which Sister commented: "A flower is a flower, but we prefer cash". In the early 1980's, facilities for Computerised Tomographic (CT) scans were scarce. On one occasion, a child in urgent need of a CT scan was sent to a private hospital and a bundle of money appeared from the safe and was given to the parents. Sister Aquinas was overheard talking to the radiologist over the phone: "Can you give us a discount?" Ward rounds were always conducted in a spirit of professionalism and good humour, and former patients were often remembered by name. Although she met Her Majesty the Queen and a number of world leaders she remained humble, but her own fame was considerable. On one occasion, a letter arrived on her desk delivered by the Post Office, addressed only to "Sister Aquinas, China".

She died peacefully on 28th November 1985 at Ruttonjee Sanatorium after a relatively brief illness . On the day before her death, she invited all the staff of the Sanatorium to visit her to say farewell, which we all did, in single file. It was a gesture typical of her outstanding personality.

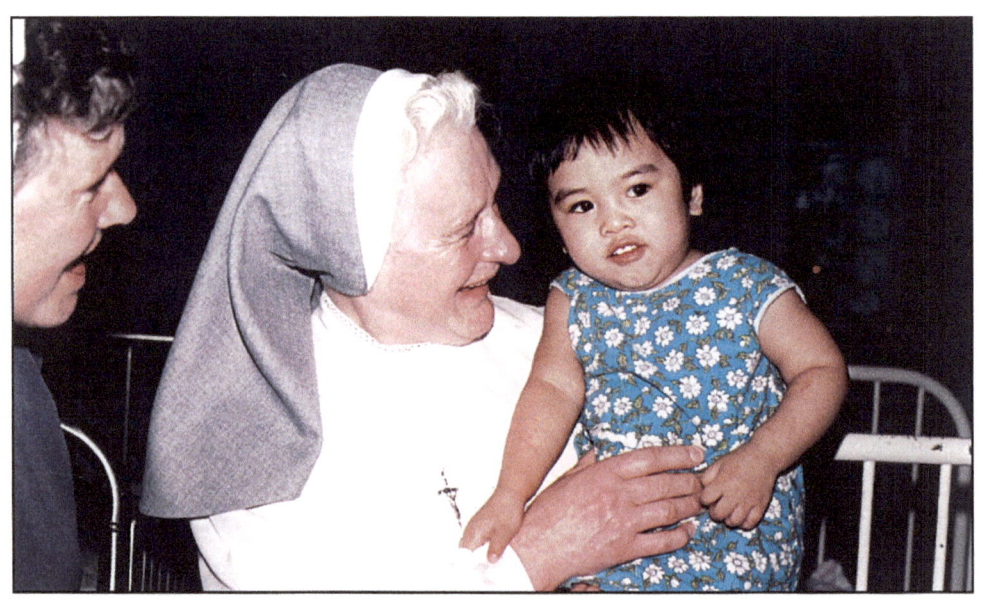

Childhood tuberculosis is now very rare in Hong Kong.

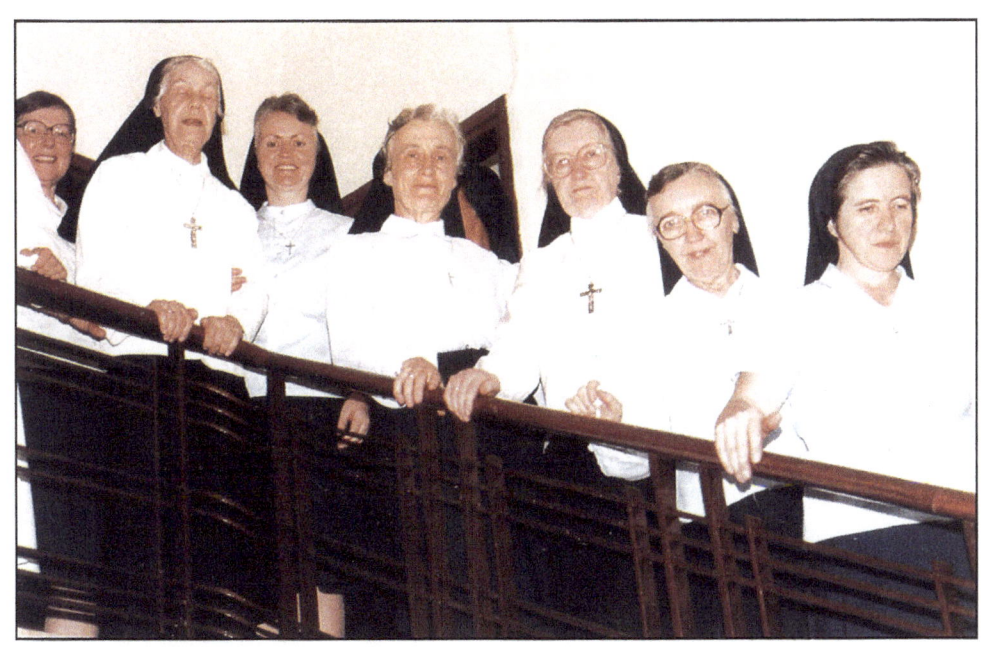

Sisters of the Order of Saint Columban provided dedicated service to the Sanatorium from 1948 to 1988.

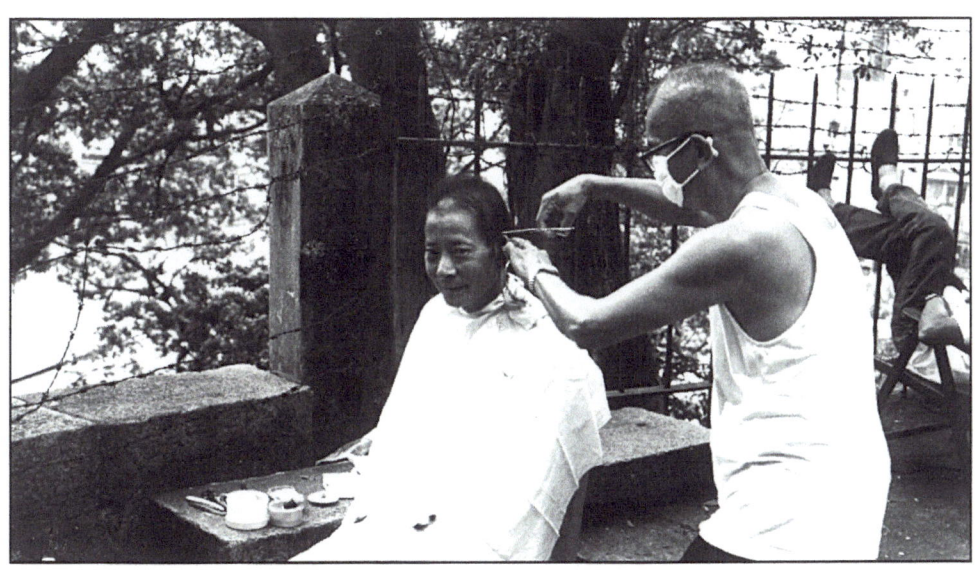

Sanatorium life: A barber visited patients on a regular basis.

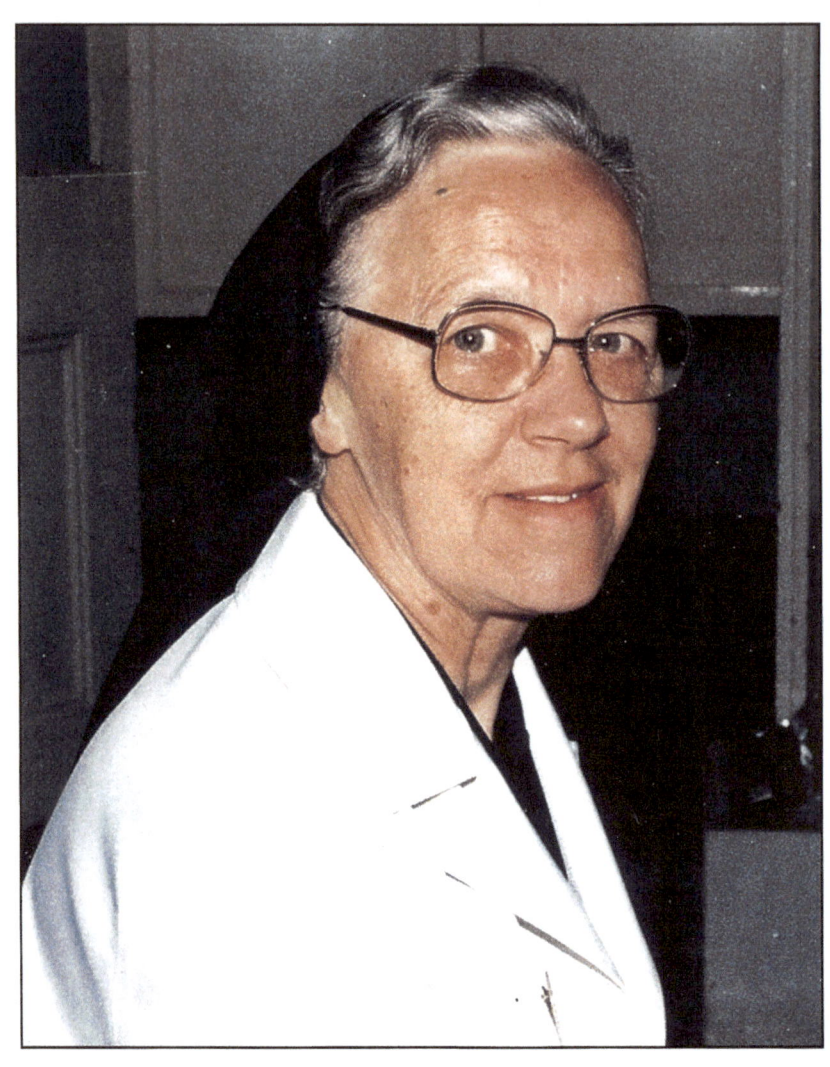

Sister Mary Gabriel, MBE, FRCP.
Physician at Ruttonjee Sanatorium from 1950 to 1988.

SISTER MARY GABRIEL

Sister Mary Gabriel, (Mary O'Mahoney) MBE, FRCP, graduated in medicine from University College, Dublin, in 1947. She served as an Intern at the Carney Hospital and at Boston City Hospital in the USA in 1949-50 and joined the medical staff of the Ruttonjee Sanatorium in 1950. Together with Sister Aquinas and the other Sisters, they established a formidable team.

As well as being a dedicated clinician, Sister Gabriel is also widely published, having special interests in asthma and allergy[48-51], childhood tuberculosis[52-54] and orthopaedic and spinal tuberculosis[55,56], collaborating with the MRC Working Party on Tuberculosis of the Spine[57-59]. During a sabattical taken at the Department of Immunology at the Brompton Hospital, laboratory techniques were developed for measuring serum antibodies to the anti-tuberculosis drug, rifampicin. This work developed into studies of the relationship of rifampicin antibodies to side-effects in daily and intermittent chemotherapy regimens, and led to a number of important publications[60-62]. However, Sister Gabriel's greatest interest was in tuberculous meningitis and, in 1973, a dedicated ward was established to care for such patients. The disease had a terrible prognosis, drugs were scarce and many patients, mostly children, were admitted unconscious. Sister Gabriel dedicated herself to their care and recruited the assistance of neurosurgeons, initially from private practice by Drs. Edmund Cheung and Peter Wu who gave their services free, and later from Queen Mary Hospital. Air encephalography and ventricular drainage were performed, where appropriate. However, the outlook for these children brightened with the advent of new anti-tuberculosis drugs such as isoniazid and streptomycin, appropriate neurosurgical intervention, and intensive nursing care.

There were a number of publications correlating clinical presentation and outcome[63-65], and more recently there were contributions concerning cerebrospinal fluid pharmacokinetics[66,67], CT scan findings[68], intracranial tuberculoma[69,70], advances in diagnosis[71] and clinical features,[72] including a review of 21 years of experience of children with tuberculous meningitis[73]. The clinical care of the patients with meningitis was further supported by Dr. Robert Teoh, Senior Lecturer in Neurology at the Chinese University of Hong Kong, who visited patients weekly on an honorary basis. Sister Gabriel retired from the Sanatorium in 1988, and was admitted as a Member of the British Empire in 1990. Recently, her energies have focused on the Society for the Promotion of Hospice Care, and the construction of a dedicated facility to care for the terminally ill, the Bradbury Hospice, which opened in June 1992.

During their time at the Sanatorium, the Sisters earned a reputation for exemplary medical and nursing care. In the field of chest diseases and tuberculosis, they contributed significantly to teaching and research, and published more than 100 scientific papers, earning international recognition for their work.

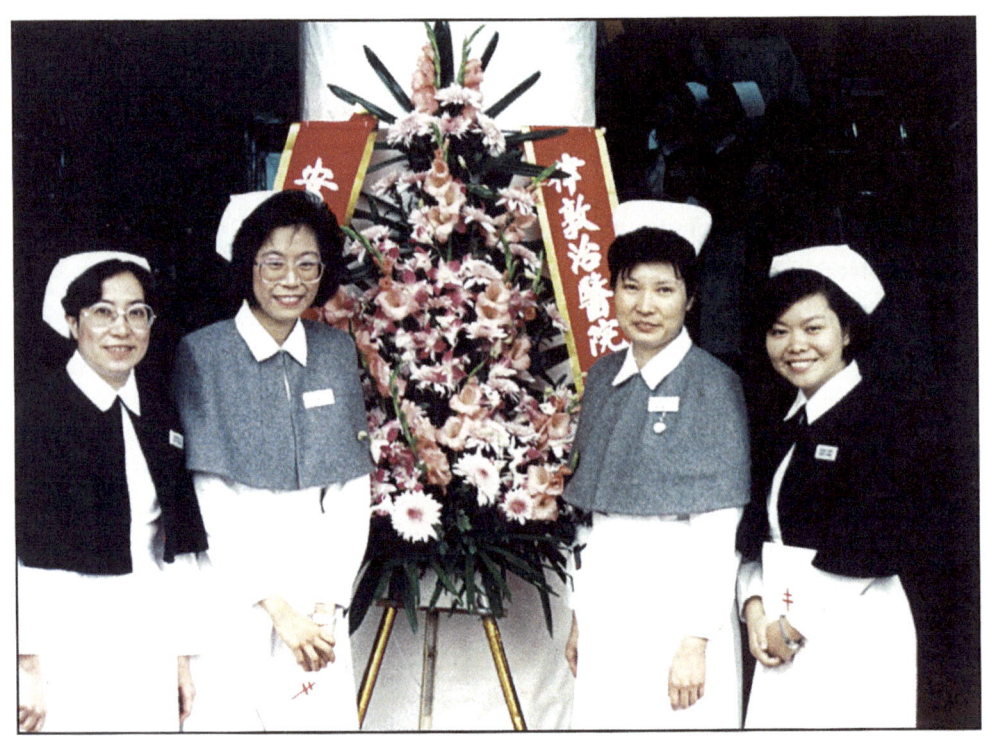

Awaiting the arrival of the Governor, Sir David Wilson, for the foundation stone laying ceremony, November 14th 1988.

The Ruttonjee Hospital

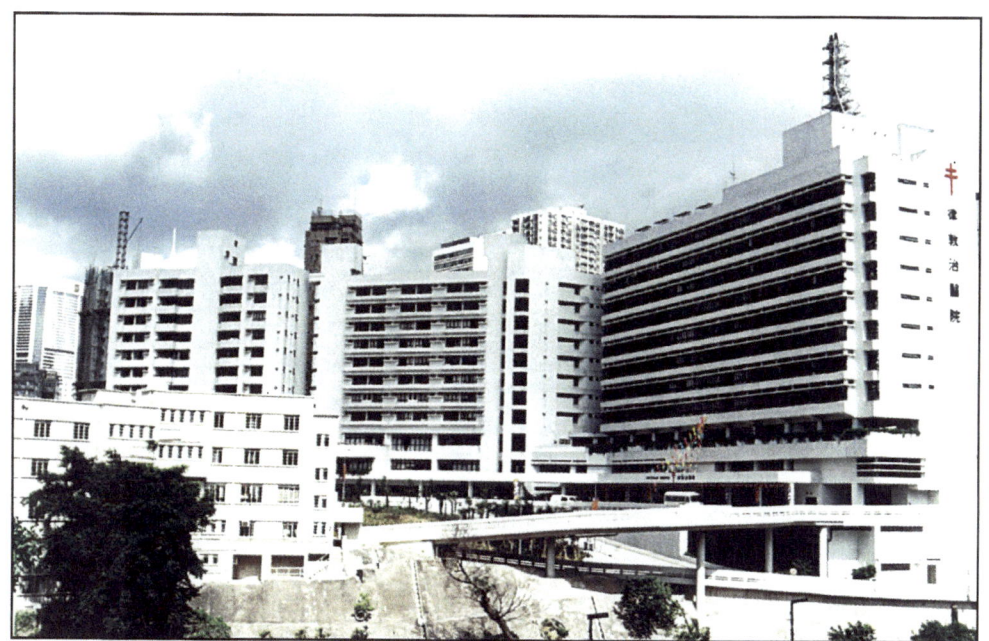

The new Ruttonjee Hospital, facing Queen's Road East, Wanchai.

In 1979, the Board of Directors decided that with the rapid increase in the population of Hong Kong, the aim of the Association and Ruttonjee Sanatorium would be to widen the scope of medical services to the public. The new Ruttonjee Hospital was planned under the Redevelopment and House Committee headed by Mr. Tseng Cheng who also donated generously towards the redevelopment project. In the garden of the Sanatorium site, the building of a 650-bed general hospital commenced in 1986 and was completed by 1990. The new hospital has general medical and surgical units, a geriatric unit, infirmary beds, a tuberculosis and chest diseases unit, and modern equipment and facilities, including a CT scanner, offering a comprehensive medical service for the people of Hong Kong. On April 22nd 1994, the Ruttonjee Hospital was officially opened by the Governor of Hong Kong, the Right Honourable Christopher Patten.

Although on the decline, tuberculosis remains an important cause of morbidity and mortality in Hong Kong. In 1994, there were 6319 new notifications (a rate of 104 per 100,000 population) and 409 deaths. Clearly there remains much work to be done.

BIBLIOGRAPHY

1. Preston P J. Medicine in Colonial Hong Kong, 1985.
2. Choa G H. The life and times of Sir Kai Ho Kai. Chinese University Press, Hong Kong 1981.
3. Harland K. The Royal Navy in Hong Kong. Maritime Books, Liskeard, 1981.
4. Eitel E J. Europe in China: The history of Hong Kong from the beginning to the year 1882. Kelly and Walsh, Hong Kong, 1895.
5. Choa G H. 'Heal the Sick' was their motto - the Protestant medical missionaries in China. Chinese University Press, Hong Kong, 1990.
6. Rydings H A. Transactions of the China Medico-Chirurgical Society 1845-6. Journal of the Hong Kong Branch of the Royal Asiatic Society 1973;13:13-27.
7. Pottinger H. Letter to Lord Stanley. Colonial Office (CO) Records 1843;(25):369-376. Public Record Office, London.
8. Harland W. Colonial Surgeon's Report for 1848, Hong Kong.
9. Harland W. Colonial Surgeon's Report for 1849, Hong Kong.
10. Admiralty Records (ADM 125/81) 1858; 231. Public Record Office, London.
11. Admiralty Records (ADM 125/19) 1873; 152-163. Public Record Office, London.
12. Admiralty Records (ADM 125/19) 1872; 148. Public Record Office, London.
13. History of the Second World War. The Royal Naval Medical Service. Vol II. Operations. Ed Coulter J L S. HMSO, London 1954.
14. Hui K L, Gabriel M. Resection in the treatment of pulmonary tuberculosis in Hong Kong. Tubercle 1962;43:361-366.
15. Hui K L, Gabriel M. Surgical treatment of pulmonary tuberculosis in Hong Kong. Pacific Med & Surg 1965;73:1-4.

16. Hodgson A R, Stock E E, Fang H S Y, Ong G B. Anterior spinal fusion. The operative approach and pathological findings in 412 patients with Pott's disease of the spine. Brit J Surgery 1960;XLVIII(208):172-178.

17. Hong Kong Tuberculosis Treatment Services/The Research Committee of the British Tuberculosis Association. A controlled trial of ethionamide with isoniazid in the treatment of pulmonary tuberculosis in Hong Kong. Tubercle 1964;45:299-320.

18. Hong Kong Tuberculosis Treatment Services/Brompton Hospital/British Medical Research Council. A controlled trial of daily and intermittent regimens plus ethambutol in the re-treatment of patients with pulmonary tuberculosis in Hong Kong. Tubercle 1974;55:1-27

19. Hong Kong Chest Service/British Medical Research Council. Controlled trial of 6-month and 9-month regimens of daily and intermittent streptomycin plus isoniazid plus pyrazinamide for pulmonary tuberculosis in Hong Kong. The results up to 30 months. Am Rev Respir Dis 1977;115:727-735.

20. Hong Kong Chest Service/British Medical Research Council. Controlled trial of 6-month and 8-month regimens in the treatment of pulmonary tuberculosis: The results up to 24 months. Tubercle 1979;60:201-210.

21. Hong Kong Chest Service/British Medical Research Council. Controlled trial of 4 three-times weekly regimens and a daily regimen all given for 6 months for pulmonary tuberculosis. Second Report: The results up to 24 months. Tubercle 1982;63:89-98.

22. Hong Kong Chest Service/British Medical Research Council. Five-year follow-up of a controlled trial of five 6-month regimens of chemotherapy for pulmonary tuberculosis. Am Rev Respir Dis 1987;136:1339-1342.

23. Hong Kong Chest Service/Tuberculosis Research Centre, Madras/British Medical Research Council. Sputum smear-negative pulmonary tuberculosis. Controlled trial of 3-month and 2-month regimens of chemotherapy. First Report. Lancet 1979;i:1361-1364.

24. Hong Kong Chest Service/Tuberculosis Research Centre, Madras/British Medical Research Council. A controlled trial of 2-month, 3-month and 12-month regimens of chemotherapy for sputum smear-negative pulmonary tuberculosis. Am Rev Respir Dis 1984;130:23-28.

25. Hong Kong Tuberculosis Treatment Services/Brompton Hospital/British Medical Research Council. A controlled trial of daily and intermittent rifampicin plus ethambutol in the re-treatment of patients with pulmonary tuberculosis. Results up to 30 months. Tubercle 1975;56:179-189.

26. Hong Kong Tuberculosis Treatment Services/British Medical Research Council. A study in Hong Kong to evaluate the role of pretreatment susceptibility tests in the selection of regimens of chemotherapy for pulmonary tuberculosis. Second Report. Tubercle 1974;55:169-192.

27. Hong Kong Tuberculosis Treatment Services/British Medical Research Council. A controlled clinical trial of small daily doses of rifampicin in the prevention of adverse reactions to the drug in a once weekly regimen of chemotherapy in Hong Kong. Second Report: The results at 12 months. Tubercle 1974;55:193-210.

28. Hong Kong Tuberculosis Treatment Services/British Medical Research Council. Investigation of allergic status and blood counts in Chinese patients receiving daily and intermittent rifampicin in Hong Kong. Clinical Allergy 1975;5:189-199.

29. Hong Kong Tuberculosis Treatment Services/British Medical Research Council. The influence of age and sex on the incidence of the 'flu' syndrome and rifampicin-dependent antibodies in patients on intermittent rifampicin for tuberculosis. Tubercle 1975;56:173-178.

30. Hong Kong Tuberculosis Treatment Services/East African/British Medical Research Council. Adverse reactions to short-course regimens containing streptomycin, isoniazid, pyrazinamide and rifampicin in Hong Kong. Tubercle 1976;57:81-95.

31. Hong Kong Chest Service/British Medical Research Council. Controlled trial of 2, 4 and 6 months of pyrazinamide in 6-month, three-times-weekly regimens for smear-positive pulmonary tuberculosis, including an assessment of a combined preparation of isoniazid, rifampicin and pyrazinamide - results at 30 months. Am Rev Respir Dis 1991;143:700-706.

32. Fox W. Compliance of patients and physicians: Experience and lessons from tuberculosis I and II. Brit Med J 1983;287:33-35, 101-5.

33. Hui K L, Aquinas M. Surgery for first line drug-resistant tuberculosis. Brit J Dis Chest 1966;49(1):57-60.

34. Aquinas M. The chronic positive patient. The Hong Kong Nursing Journal 1969;38-40.

35. Lim B T, Aquinas M. Ethambutol and capreomycin in the retreatment of advanced pulmonary tuberculosis. Am Rev Respir Dis 1969;99:792-793.

36. Aquinas M, Citron K M. Rifampicin, ethambutol and capreomycin in pulmonary tuberculosis, previously treated with both first and second-line drugs: The results of 2 years chemotherapy. Tubercle 1972;53:153-165.

37. Aquinas M. Rifampicin, ethambutol and capreomycin in pulmonary tuberculosis, previously treated with standard and reserve regimens: The results four years later. Bull Hong Kong Med Assoc 1973;25:61-64.

38. Aquinas M. Reactions to anti-tuberculosis drugs among Chinese in Hong Kong. Tubercle 1964;45(3):181-187.

39. Aquinas M, Allan W G L, Jenkins P K, Wong H Y, Girling D, Tall R, Fox W. Adverse reactions to daily and intermittent rifampicin regimens for pulmonary tuberculosis in Hong Kong. Brit Med J 1972;(1):765-771.

40. Aquinas M. Adverse reactions to daily and intermittent rifampicin and their management. Symposium proceedings, Rifampicin and current policies in antituberculosis chemotherapy. CIBA 1972;75-85.

41. Aquinas M. Pyrazinamide and ethionamide in the treatment of pulmonary tuberculosis in Hong Kong. Tubercle 1963;44(1):76-81.

42. Aquinas M. Drug treatment of pulmonary tuberculosis. Medical Progress 1974;27-31.
43. Aquinas M. Observations on controlled clinical trials for tuberculosis in Hong Kong. Bull Hong Kong Med Assoc 1974;26:31-37.
44. Aquinas M. Changing concepts in tuberculosis control. Soc Comm Med Hong Kong Bull 1977;8:64-85.
45. Aquinas M. The control of tuberculosis in Hong Kong. Bull Hong Kong Assoc Pharm 1979;20:3-5.
46. Aquinas M. The prevalence of tuberculin sensitivity and its relation to a BCG vaccination program among Chinese in Hong Kong. Am Rev Tuberc and Pulm Dis 1957;76(2):215-224.
47. Aquinas M, Todd D. Particular problems of tuberculosis in developing countries. Oxford Textbook of Medicine 1987; 5.262-5.267. Oxford.
48. Gabriel M, Allen W G L, Hill L E, Nunn A J. Study of prolonged hyposensitization with D. pteronyssinus extract in allergic rhinitis. Clinical Allergy 1977;7:325-336.
49. Gabriel M, Wong C, Viner A S. A study of 2% solution of sodium cromoglycate (Lomusol) in Hong Kong Chinese. Bull Hong Kong Med Assoc 1978;30:13-19.
50. Gabriel M, Ng H K, Allan W G L. Allergic rhinitis treated by intranasal beclomethasone diproprionate. Mod Med Asia 1980;16(5):36-39.
51. Gabriel M, Cunnington A M, Allan W G L, Pickering C A C, Wraith D G. Mite allergy in Hong Kong. Clinical Allergy 1982;12:157-171.
52. Gabriel M. Treatment of tuberculosis in childhood. J Paeds, Obs & Gynae 1981;41-46.
53. Gabriel M. Pulmonary tuberculosis in childhood. J Paeds Obs & Gynae 1986;17-22.
54. Sham M K, Humphries M J, Gabriel M. Childhood respiratory tuberculosis in Hong Kong - A study of 301 children with respiratory tuberculosis treated at Ruttonjee Sanatorium 1980-1986 inclusive. Hong Kong J Paediatr 1989;6:3-8.

55. Hodgson A R, Smith T K, Gabriel M. Tuberculosis of the wrist. Clin Orthop 1972;83:73-83.

56. Bailey H, Gabriel M, Hodgson A R D, Shin J S. Tuberculosis of the spine in children. Operative findings and results in one hundred consecutive patients treated by removal of the lesion and anterior grafting. J Bone & Joint Surg (Am) 1972;54:1633-1657.

57. Fourth report of the Medical Research Council Working Party on Tuberculosis of the Spine. A controlled trial of anterior spinal fusion and debridement in the surgical management of tuberculosis of the spine in patients on standard chemotherapy: A study in Hong Kong. Brit J Surg 1974;61:853-866.

58. Sixth Report of the Medical Research Council Working Party on Tuberculosis of the Spine. Five-year assessment of controlled trials of ambulatory treatment, debridement and anterior spinal fusion in the management of tuberculosis of the spine. Studies in Bulawayo (Rhodesia) and in Hong Kong. Bone & Joint Surg 1978;60(2):163-177.

59. Tenth report of the Medical Research Council Working Party on Tuberculosis of the Spine. A controlled trial of six-month and nine-month regimens of chemotherapy in patients undergoing radical surgery for tuberculosis of the spine in Hong Kong. Tubercle 1986;67:243-259.

60. Gabriel M. Observations on antibody reaction scores on individual patients. Scand J Resp Dis 1973;84:64-72.

61. Gabriel M, Chew W K. Relationship between rifampicin - dependent antibody scores, serum rifampicin concentrations and symptoms in patients with adverse reactions to intermittent rifampicin treatment. Clinical Allergy 1973;3:353-362.

62. Dickinson J M, Mitchison D A, Lee S K, Ong Y Y, Gabriel M, Girling D, Nunn A J. Serum rifampicin concentrations related to dose size and to the incidence of the 'flu' syndrome during intermittent rifampicin administration. J Antimicrob Chemother 1977;3:445-452.

63. Gabriel M, Howlett G, Lui W Y. Tuberculous Meningitis. Bull Hong Kong Med Assoc 1975;27:55-65.

64. Gabriel M. Tuberculous Meningitis in Hong Kong. Symposium Proceedings. CIBA 1979.

65. Girling D, Darbyshire J, Humphries M J, Gabriel M. Tuberculous meningitis. In "Extrapulmonary Tuberculosis". Brit Med Bull 1988;44(3):738-756.

66. Ellard G A, Humphries M J, Gabriel M, Teoh R. Penetration of pyrazinamide into the cerebrospinal fluid in tuberculous meningitis. Brit Med J 1987;294:284-285.

67. Woo J, Humphries M J, Chan K, O'Mahoney G, Teoh R. Cerebrospinal fluid and serum levels of pyrazinamide and rifampicin in patients with tuberculous meningitis. Curr Ther Res 1987;42(2):236-242.

68. Teoh R, Humphries M J, Hoare R D, O'Mahoney G. Clinical correlation of CT changes in 64 patients with tuberculous meningitis. J Neurol 1989;236:48-51.

69. Teoh R, Humphries M J, O'Mahoney G. Symptomatic intracranial tuberculoma developing during treatment for tuberculosis. A report of ten patients and review of the literature. Quart J Med 1987;241:449-460.

70. Teoh R, Poon W, Humphries M J, O'Mahoney G. Suprasellar tuberculoma developing during treatment of tuberculous meningitis requiring urgent surgical decompression. J Neurol 1988;235:321-322.

71. French G L, Teoh R, Chan C Y, Humphries M J, Cheung S W, O'Mahoney G. Diagnosis of tuberculous meningitis by detection of tuberculostearic acid in cerebrospinal fluid. Lancet 1987;ii:117-119.

72. Teoh R, Humphries M J, Chan J C N, Ng H K, O'Mahony G. Internuclear ophthalmoplegia in tuberculous meningitis. Tubercle 1989;70:61-64.

73. Humphries M J, Teoh R, Lau J, Gabriel M. Factors of prognostic significance in Chinese children with tuberculous meningitis. Tubercle 1990;71:161-168

Appendix A

Letter to the Right Honorable Lord Stanley from Sir Henry Pottinger, Governor, dated November 28th 1843, Victoria, Hong Kong.

I have begged Lord Aberdeen to furnish your Lordship with a copy of my Dispatch No. 152 of the 20th instant, on the subject of the Seamen's Hospital which has been established in this Colony, chiefly through the means of a donation of $12,000, made by Mr. Heerjeebhoy Rustomjee, and for the site of which hospital I granted a piece of ground so long ago as February 1842.

I received a further application asking me to allot the Marine Lots surrounding the Hill on which the hospital is built (and which overlooks the harbour) for the support of the institution, but I have hitherto not contributed in any shape, beyond the piece of ground for the site of the building.

The two letters on this subject are numbered 4 and 56, of the February 22nd and the April 30th 1842 and will be found in the 1st Volume of the Colonial Outwards Correspondence which I forwarded to your Lordship by Lieut-Colonel Malcolm.

The support of the present hospital is one of those questions regarding which it is impossible to say whether it belongs most strictly to the Department of the Government of this Colony, or to that of Her Majesty's Chief Superintendent of Trade but the extension of its' advantages and uses, as described in the accompanying copy of a letter dated the 25th Instant, which has been addressed to me by Mr. Anderson - the Colonial Surgeon - clearly appertains to the Colony; and I have, therefore, thought it right to submit that letter for your Lordship's information and commands.

It is needless for me to occupy your Lordship's time by enlarging on the necessity for such an institution in this Colony, although there is not now time to prepare the details spoken of in the concluding passage of Mr. Anderson's letter. I, therefore, at present, only think it right to respectfully recommend for your Lordship's favourable consideration that Her Majesty's Government may grant a sum at least equal to the donation of Mr. Heerjeebhoy Rustomjee, to increase the building and also a monthly allowance of two hundred dollars to keep up the requisite establishments, as well as to provide medicines, hospital furniture &c, &c.

When the whole of this monthly allowance may not be expended, I would propose, that the balance should be carried to the credit of the "Hospital Fund"; that the expenditure should be audited, once a quarter, by a Committee (of which the Colonial Surgeon and one or two other Officers of Government should be ex-officio members) and submitted to the Governor in Council for fund sanction, and that defined rules as to the admission of patients, the stoppages (where they were in the pay of the Government) to be made from these patients, and other requisite details should be framed and promulgated under the same authority and sanction.

Should it be thought advisable, hereafter, to meet the expenses of both the Seamen's and General Hospitals by appropriating to that object, the rents accruing from Marine Lots situated in the immediate neighbourhood of the hospitals - a plan which is alluded to in one of the letters already quoted - there is no doubt but this might be done. I am however, disposed to think that a fixed monthly allowance be paid from the Colonial Treasury would be better, as ensuring perfect regularity, and obviating any risk of a failure in the pecuniary resources of the Institution from locations not being tenanted, or other similar causes.

It is perhaps proper I should acquaint your Lordship that a member of the public servants of the inferior grades (Police, Road Overseers &c, &c) of Government, have been necessarily sent to the Hospital, even on its present footing, during the late unhealthy season, and have received gratuitous professional attendance from the Gentlemen who devote themselves to that humane and charitable purpose; but who could not spare time to visit the sick at their usual residences, so that, to a certain extent, the plans pointed out by Mr. Anderson have had a trial, and this has been found to answer every useful and convenient purpose.

APPENDIX B

Letter to the Right Honourable W. E. Gladstone MP, from Sir John F. Davis; Governor and Commander-in-Chief, dated April 15th 1846, Victoria, Hong Kong.

The most gratifying subject of the present Report is the successful vindication of the colony from those charges of unhealthiness, which accidental circumstances (some of them inseperably connected with its first occupation) swelled into a species of panic about the time I quitted England, and led many persons to imagine that a residence in the place was a desperate undertaking. Some unprincipled attempts were made (even after the truth was known) to augment this panic, by the most elaborate misrepresentations, and a great deal of nonsense about 'decayed granite' etc, but the best answer, on the whole, is the remarkable immunity from disease which followed immediately upon the completion of fitting dwellings, efficient drainage and other improvements.

The delightful winter which prevails here will, I have no doubt, make Hong Kong a place of resort to invalids from India. The Colonial Surgeon's very complete Report at pages 127-138 of the Blue Book will be found amply to corroborate the above statement, and to prove that this Colony is much more healthy than many others of Her Majesty's inter-tropical possessions. Even in the case of the Troops (by no means an infallible test of climate) the mortality was reduced to nearly a half during the last year, before their present excellent barracks were completed; and now that the soldiers have been housed in them, I entertain no doubt of the marked and favourable result.

www.ingramcontent.com/pod-product-compliance
Lightning Source LLC
Chambersburg PA
CBHW040840180526
45159CB00001B/261